A LIFELONG DIET PLAN TO REDUCE YOUR RISK OF CANCER!

The cancer statistics are terrifying, but now, for the first time, the National Academy of Science has released information pointing to how they can be significantly reversed.

Studies have shown that what you eat and drink, and how *much* you eat and drink of certain things, can actually increase—or reduce—your risk of getting cancer. This means that THE LIFELONG ANTI-CANCER DIET can be the most important diet of your life. All that it requires of you is that you become aware of high-risk foods and cancer-prevention foods, and eat accordingly.

This breakthrough book provides all the anti-cancer facts about foods and vitamins, as well as recipes and menu suggestions. It is the simplest ever, easiest-to-stay-with, lifelong plan to save your health and the health of your loved ones—

THE LIFELONG ANTI-CANCER DIET

D1560207

SIGNET Books for Your Reference Shelf

THE LIFELONG ANTI-CANCER DIET

Carmel Berman Reingold

With a Foreword by
Edward Essner, Ph.D.

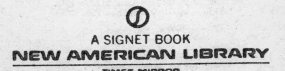

A SIGNET BOOK
NEW AMERICAN LIBRARY
TIMES MIRROR

PUBLISHER'S NOTE

The ideas, procedures, and suggestions contained in this book are
not intended as a substitute for consulting with your physician. All
matters regarding your health require medical supervision.

NAL BOOKS ARE AVAILABLE AT QUANTITY DISCOUNTS WHEN USED TO PROMOTE
PRODUCTS OR SERVICES. FOR INFORMATION PLEASE WRITE TO PREMIUM
MARKETING DIVISION, THE NEW AMERICAN LIBRARY, INC., 1633 BROADWAY,
NEW YORK, NEW YORK 10019.

SIGNET TRADEMARK REG. U.S. PAT. OFF. AND FOREIGN COUNTRIES
REGISTERED TRADEMARK—MARCA REGISTRADA
HECHO EN CHICAGO, U.S.A.

SIGNET, SIGNET CLASSICS, MENTOR, PLUME, MERIDIAN and NAL BOOKS
are published by The New American Library, Inc.,
1633 Broadway, New York, New York 10019

First Printing, November, 1982

1 2 3 4 5 6 7 8 9

PRINTED IN THE UNITED STATES OF AMERICA

CONTENTS

ACKNOWLEDGMENTS

I would like to thank the consultants who spent their valuable time clarifying scientific data, and who were constantly encouraging in their appraisal of this project:

Dr. Edward Essner, cell biologist, member of the American Association for Cancer Research, member of the American Society for Cell Biology. Dr. Essner worked in cancer research at the National Cancer Institute and at Sloan-Kettering Institute. He is presently at Wayne State University, Michigan.

Dr. Norman J. Levy, psychiatrist, psychoanalyst, physician. Dr. Levy is a member of the American Academy of Psychoanalysis, and is on the staff of the Post-Graduate Center for Mental Health in New York City.

Dr. Abraham O. Zoss, Fellow of the American Association for the Advancement of Science, a member of the New York Academy of Sciences, and a Fellow of the American Institute of Chemists.

My thanks, too, to Ms. Gail Piazza, nutritionist, and to Ms. Susan David, Library of Congress.

FOREWORD

Diet, Nutrition, and Cancer, the report recently issued by a committee appointed by the National Academy of Sciences, was the heuristic medium that inspired *The Lifelong Anti-Cancer Diet*.

This latter work is a serious and scrupulous explanation of the committee's findings relative to diet and cancer, and both the background and the basis of those findings are clearly defined.

The Lifelong Anti-Cancer Diet can be easily followed, and the moderate and considered counsels of this work act as both concrete example and model of the dietary guidelines recommended in the report issued by the National Academy of Sciences.

The Lifelong Anti-Cancer Diet explains how the nutritional guidelines and dietary recommendations that were an intrinsic part of the original work can now be comprehensively applied to our daily lives.

—*Dr. Edward Essner*

PREFACE

Both my parents died of cancer at a relatively young age, and according to some scientific studies, this means that I am genetically primed to have cancer at some time in my life, too.

Of course, no one knows for sure. There is much that is unknown about a disease that has more than a hundred forms. There does seem to be a family tendency toward cancer. Is there a lack of immunity programmed within the genes? Possibly. Possibly, too, there is a tendency of family members to live alike, and follow the same habits that might increase the risks of cancer. I did smoke, but I no longer do so. Both my parents smoked, but watching them die made me give up the habit.

My parents, not normally given to fooling themselves, certainly fooled themselves when it came to smoking. Everyone now knows about the connection between tobacco and cancer.

Now we're learning that certain diets—certain ways of eating—can also increase the risks of cancer. Does it make sense for me to ignore that information? Shouldn't I, therefore, be more aware of the way I eat? And I speak not only for myself, but for the people I love, the people I lovingly cook for, and the ones I may be helping to destroy with my overly rich, overly loving cooking.

Dr. Clifford Grobstein, Professor of Biological Science at the University of California and chairman of the National Academy of Sciences committee that prepared the eye-opening report *Diet, Nutrition, and Cancer* said, "It is time to further spread the message that cancer is not as inevitable as death and taxes."

The panel of scientists working with Dr. Grobstein presented specific dietary guidelines. If these guidelines can lessen the risk of cancer, wouldn't it be foolish not to follow them?

When I decided to write this book I called my good friend Dr. Edward Essner, a scientist and presently a professor at Wayne State University in Michigan. Dr. Essner had worked in cancer research for years at the National Cancer Institute and at Sloan-Kettering Institute, and he has been the unfortunate recipient through the years of my various calls announcing the cancer illness of someone I loved and asking for advice as to the "best" doctor to see, the "best" hospital to go to, the "best" specialist to consult regarding a particular type of cancer.

When I called this time, the worry in Dr. Essner's voice was apparent. No one was ill, I assured him. I wanted to consult him about the recent study linking cancer and diet. It was nice, for a change, to talk about the hopeful possibility of preventing cancer.

This book is for my mother and my father, and my good friend Jack Pacey, and my cousin Dezsö David, beloved victims all.

CHAPTER ONE

THE BASIS OF THE LIFELONG ANTI-CANCER DIET PLAN

If you were told that you could greatly reduce the risk of cancer by doing nothing more difficult than following a plan of diet and nutrition based on a scientific study, would you do it?

Of course, you might have to eliminate certain favorite foods, and cut down on others. It would also be important to add other foods rich in specific vitamins and nutrients that are known to reduce the risk of cancer. But this is all you would have to do. You wouldn't be required to buy anything expensive or exotic. You might even save money. Everything on this diet plan would be readily available.

You've probably tried many diets before, mostly to lose weight, to look better. Wouldn't you be willing now to try a diet that can reduce the risk of cancer?

THE GOOD NEWS

But is there such a diet? Is there a way of eating that can actually reduce the risk of some cancers? The breathtakingly good news is that there is!

For the very first time an expert committee of the National Academy of Sciences has conducted an exten-

1

sive study exploring the possibility of a link between diet and cancer.

The committee began its work in 1980, when the National Cancer Institute commissioned the National Research Council of the National Academy of Sciences to do a comprehensive study of all available scientific information concerning the relationship of diet and nutrition to cancer. A committee was formed, and the members represented such disciplines as biochemistry, microbiology, embryology, epidemiology, experimental oncology, internal medicine, microbial genetics, molecular biology, molecular genetics, nutrition, nutrition education, public health, and toxicology.

The committee, whose diverse disciplines were able to provide a broad perspective as well as comprehensive coverage of the subject, examined both epidemiological studies and laboratory studies to determine the possibility of a relationship between diet and cancer.

The result of the committee's study is a report entitled *Diet, Nutrition and Cancer*. The National Academy of Sciences has recently released that report, which does indicate a definite link between cancer and nutrition. According to the panel of scientists, what we eat, how much of our chosen foods we eat, and what we drink can actually increase—or reduce—the risk of cancer. As they stated:

"By some estimates, as much as 90% of all cancer in humans has been attributed to various environmental factors, including diet. . . . investigators have estimated that diet is responsible for 30% to 40% of cancers in men and 60% of cancers in women. Recently, two epidemiologists suggested that a significant proportion of the deaths from cancer could be prevented by dietary means. . . ."

THE LIFELONG DIET PLAN

The Lifelong Anti-Cancer Diet, which is explained in detail later on in this book, follows the committee's dietary recommendations and guidelines. There is also a 21-Day Menu Plan which illustrates how you can apply this important body of scientific knowledge to the way you eat, and to the meals prepared for yourself and your family. In addition to menus, there is important nutritional information for each meal, as well as recipes to help meal planning easier.

CHAPTER TWO

NUTRITION: THE BIG BREAKTHROUGH

"It is highly likely that the United States will eventually have the option of adopting a diet that reduces its incidence of cancer by approximately one-third," according to the National Research Council's report.

The chairman of the committee, Dr. Clifford Grobstein, also said, "The evidence is increasingly impressive that what we eat does affect our chances of getting cancer. This is good news, because it means that by controlling what we eat, we may prevent such diet-sensitive cancers."

All of us would like to hear that the scientists who worked on the report said that proper diet *positively*, *definitely* can prevent cancers. Instead they use the word *may*, but there's a hefty body of scientific evidence behind that word *may*. It's important to remember that twenty years ago the Surgeon General released a report stating that "cigarettes *may* cause cancer."

Today we know that there's no *may* about it. Cigarettes are the cause of just about one-quarter of all the fatal cancers in the United States.

That early report on cigarette smoking was considered an interim report, as is this report linking diet to cancer. There are no guarantees—just as when you hear a television weather report saying "sunny and fair tomorrow" there are no guarantees that the forecaster will be 100% right. He probably will be, because he's based his forecast on expertly gathered data.

The probability that the report linking diet to cancer is accurate is also very high. The body of scientific knowledge accumulated through years of research offers impressive proof, and the correlation of facts and figures is startling.

The report contains hard facts and figures. Ignoring them, in an ostrichlike fashion, would be foolhardy, and could be dangerous.

There is no good reason why sitting down to breakfast, lunch, or dinner should be the equivalent of a death-defying act—not when there are possible and pleasant alternatives. And when we know that approximately 20% of all deaths in the United States are caused by cancer it would be frivolous to say, "I'll take my chances that it won't be me."

According to the American Cancer Society's "1982 Cancer Facts & Figures" as well as statistics from other sources:

About 58 million Americans now living will eventually have cancer.

One out of four people will eventually have cancer at present rates, but because cancer is on the increase, this proportion may rise to three out of ten people.

An estimated 1,235,000 new cases of cancer will be diagnosed in the United States in 1982, and at this time, one person dies of cancer every 73 seconds.

At this rate, there may not be a single family that will remain untouched and unscarred by the tragedy of cancer.

Some chances in life must be taken. But risking our lives because of what we eat is too trivial to contemplate—not once we know that we have a choice.

Does this mean that all cancers can be prevented by knowledgeable nutrition? Unfortunately, no. There are other causes of cancer. Smoking greatly increases the chance of lung cancer, for example, as does living in an area where improper disposal of toxic wastes pollutes the environment. Some cancers may be caused by incompletely understood viruses or by lowered immunological defenses. But as the report stated, proper diet could reduce cancer by about one-third, which means that close to *20 million lives could be saved from cancer* by following dietary guidelines. One of those may be your life—or the life of someone you love.

How did the scientists come to the conclusion that many cancers are linked to what we eat?

The study revealed an exciting, eye-opening fact:

Types of cancer vary from country to country. When people emigrate to another country they no longer contract the cancers they might have gotten in the land of their birth. If they get cancer, it is a type prevalent in their adopted land.

People from Africa and Japan, for example, who move to the United States are afflicted with cancers typical to the United States, and atypical for Africa and Japan.

The reason? Diet! When people move to another country and live there for a while, they change the way they eat. Their food preferences become those of their new home, and these new dietary habits are reflected in the types of cancer incurred.

Once they understood the close correlation between diet and cancer, the scientists could say, " . . . the differences in the rates at which various cancers occur in different human populations are often correlated with differences in diet. . . . it has become clear that most cancers have external causes, and in principle, should therefore be preventable.''

How did the scientists decide that some cancers could be prevented? Their task was long and laborious. They knew that the richer a country, the greater the risk of cancer of the breast, colon, and uterus, but they didn't know why. They had to search out the reasons, had to discover if some or any part of the diet of an affluent society increased the risk of those particular cancers.

Working over a period of years, scientists studied various groups of people in the United States, including those who came here from other countries. Slowly, a pattern emerged:

People whose diets were loaded with fats or with a great deal of salt-cured, salt-pickled, and smoked foods, for example, had a greater incidence of certain cancers.

Other people who had low-fat diets and preferred certain fruits and vegetables had a lower incidence of those same cancers.

The research connecting cancer and diet was conducted both in and out of laboratories. Once scientists had the information that certain dietary habits seemed to increase the risk of certain cancers, while other dietary patterns tended to reduce them, they then analyzed in minute detail the various components of certain foods in order to further unravel the mystery linking nutrition to cancer.

Scientists around the world worked long and patiently to unravel the pattern linking diet to cancer, and what follows are ten potentially lifesaving discoveries that they've made.

LIFESAVING DISCOVERY #1:
Fats

Americans diet by the millions, and according to many different programs—some have gone on body-maintenance schedules that have not been seen since Empress Elizabeth was the ruling glamour girl of the Hapsburg Austro-Hungarian Empire. But the emphasis has been on diet for good looks, for cosmetic reasons, for a youthful appearance. Perhaps now the emphasis will switch to diet for life and health.

What's the difference? If thin is good, what's the difference in how you get there? The difference is that too many of us try to remain slim by crash-dieting for five days, and then eating fat-filled foods for the next two. We feel entitled to a reward, and we don't realize that the reward can be dangerous.

At this time, scientists are not sure if a large consumption of calories—any and all kinds—is linked to cancer. It's possible, but all the evidence is not yet in.

But what is known is that a high rate of cancer of the breast, large bowel, and prostate often goes along with a high rate of fat consumption. This isn't the final word, but enough data indicate such a correlation.

LIFESAVING DISCOVERY #2:
Vitamin A

Do you remember all those times your mother told you to eat all your carrots? And how about when you were visiting Aunt Sally and Uncle Mike and they told you that if you didn't eat every bit of broccoli you wouldn't get any dessert?

The words "It's good for you" haunted many of us as children; hearing "It's good for you" was enough to make us hate whatever it was.

But we're not kids any longer, and now when scientists tell us that foods like carrots and broccoli are good for us, we'd better listen to them. These vegetables, and others such as sweet potatoes, kale, and lettuce, contain beta-carotene, which is a precursor or forerunner of Vitamin A. Beta-carotene is converted to Vitamin A in the body, and Vitamin A can reduce the risk of cancer, especially in the bladder, larynx, and lungs.

LIFESAVING DISCOVERY #3:
Vitamin C

For years now we've been told that Vitamin C can cure a cold faster, but the latest news about it is even better, because now scientists believe that Vitamin C can actually inhibit the formation of certain carcinogens— cancer-causing agents that increase the incidence of cancer.

This is only part of the wonderful Vitamin C story. There is gathering evidence linking consumption of foods rich in Vitamin C (citrus fruits, tomatoes, berries, and spinach are among them) to a lowered incidence of cancer of the stomach and the esophagus.

LIFESAVING DISCOVERY #4:
Cruciferous Vegetables

A word that's new to many of us has appeared on the scene—*cruciferous*. In botany, a cruciferous plant is one that bears a flower with a crosslike, four-petaled corolla. Broccoli, cauliflower, kale, brussels sprouts, and cabbage are cruciferous vegetables, and they are strongly linked to lowered incidence of stomach, colon, and rectal cancer.

If you hate brussels sprouts you can always eat cabbage—think of cole slaw, and stuffed cabbage rolls—and if you can't abide cauliflower there is always broccoli. The choices are many. You can enjoy your favorite cruciferous vegetable and do yourself a lot of good at the same time.

LIFESAVING DISCOVERY #5:
Salt-Cured, Salt-Pickled, and Smoked Foods, and Foods Preserved with Nitrates and Nitrites

Studies have shown that in such countries as China and Japan where people tend to eat much salt-cured and salt-pickled food there has been a greater incidence of esophagus and stomach cancer. It was further discovered that some methods of pickling and smoking foods cause cancer in animals, and could cause cancer in humans.

Knowing this, the committee recommends eating less salt-cured, salt-pickled, and smoked foods, as well as foods preserved with nitrates and nitrites. This doesn't mean that you can never, ever eat smoked salmon, smoked trout, bacon, or other smoked or pickled foods again. The advice is to keep their consumption to a minimum.

LIFESAVING DISCOVERY #6:
Smoking and Drinking

The cancer-causing effects of smoking have been known for many years, but what is news is the combined effect of drinking and smoking at the same time. It's a triple threat: (1) Smoking can cause cancer; (2) excessive drinking can cause injuries to the liver which may lead to liver cancer; and (3) heavy drinking while smoking increases the risk for mouth, lung, larynx, and esophageal cancers.

LIFESAVING DISCOVERY #7:
Taking Multi-Vitamins and Minerals as Diet Supplements

The scientists say that the best way of getting enough important vitamins and minerals is through what you eat. A Vitamin A deficiency can increase the risk of certain cancers, but an overdose of Vitamin A can be toxic, and therefore the recommendation is to eat foods that contain a balance of vitamins and minerals. Don't attempt to dominate nutrition with vitamin and mineral supplements. Little pink or yellow pills can be good, but they can also be dangerous. Absorbing nutrition from food is a much safer and more sensible cancer deterrent.

If you're enamored of dietary supplements, consider the following facts before you embark on megadose pills:

Zinc: Some studies indicate that a high level of zinc has increased cancer in certain parts of the body. Other studies show that zinc levels are lower in some cancer patients.

Iodine: Either too much or too little iodine can increase the risk of cancer of the thyroid.

Selenium: In laboratory experiments with animals, selenium has been shown to have an anti-cancer effect, but a comparatively high level of selenium for humans could be toxic.

Because it's so difficult to predict the effects of high dosages of isolated vitamins or minerals, the guidelines are based on what you eat, rather than on supplements which might have a toxic potential.

LIFESAVING DISCOVERY #8:
Iron

For years an iron deficiency was associated with anemia and a feeling of fatigue. Now an iron deficiency has been linked to an increased risk in a syndrome associated with cancer of the upper alimentary canal—the passage involved with the digestion and absorption of food. Eating iron-rich foods, such as spinach and raisins, could lessen the risk of the syndrome associated with upper alimentary cancer.

LIFESAVING DISCOVERY #9:
Vitamin E

For years, health-food enthusiasts have been attributing all kinds of benefits to Vitamin E: shiny hair, more energy, greater sexual vitality. However, because Vitamin E is present in so many foods, scientists have found it hard to define the exact effects of this vitamin.

The current report says that Vitamin E does inhibit the formation of nitrosamines—highly carcinogenic chemicals—in laboratory tests conducted both *in vitro* and *in vivo,* which means tests conducted both outside a living body, as in a glass dish or a test tube, and in a living body—within living animals.

It's easy enough to include foods rich in Vitamin E in your daily diet, because this vitamin is found in vegetable oils, whole grain cereal products, and eggs.

LIFESAVING DISCOVERY #10:
The Fruit-Vegetable Group and the
Bread-Cereals Group

Who doesn't remember the constant emphasis placed on the importance of a balanced diet?

Balance, we were told, used to mean the Four Food Groups: the dairy group, the meat-fish-egg group, the vegetable-fruit group, and the bread-cereals group.

But now we know that some of these food groups are more important than others, and "balanced diet" has come to mean something else.

"The committee emphasizes the importance of including fruits, vegetables, and whole grain cereal products in the daily diet.''

Those are the exact words taken from the report.

Does this mean that protein-rich foods should be eliminated or drastically cut down in the daily diet? Scientists say that while there might be an association between a protein-rich diet and high cancer risk, the final word is not yet in. Many high-protein foods are also high in fat, and high fat, rather than high protein, could be the culprit.

Not enough is known about the relationship of protein to cancer, but much is known about the danger of fat, and the benefits of certain fruits, vegetables, and whole grain cereal products. Therefore, today's balanced diet should take advantage of this important, documented knowledge.

CHAPTER THREE

WHAT THE LIFELONG DIET CAN MEAN TO YOU

What can the report *Diet, Nutrition and Cancer* do for you? Can it really be important to your health, and the health of your family?

The answer is a resounding yes! No diet can insure against cancer, but understanding more about the nutritional values of the foods you eat and basing your daily diet on the guidelines recommended by the committee that composed the report for the National Academy of Sciences could reduce the risk of cancer, and any information that reduces that risk may be lifesaving!

The Lifelong Anti-Cancer Diet was developed after extensive study of the *Diet, Nutrition and Cancer* report, and it incorporates the committee's dietary recommendations and guidelines regarding the foods that should be eaten in greater and lesser quantities to reduce the risk of cancer. A 21-Day Menu Plan and a group of recipes show you how, in an easy way, you can follow the committee's suggestions every day.

Consulting with me on this project were:

Dr. Edward Essner, cell biologist who worked in cancer research at the National Cancer Institute and at Sloan-Kettering Institute, and who is presently at Wayne State University in Michigan. Dr. Essner is a member of the American Society for Cell Biology and the American Association for Cancer Research.

Dr. Abraham O. Zoss, who is a Fellow of the American Association for the Advancement of Science, a member of the New York Academy of Sciences, and a Fellow of the American Institute of Chemists.

Dr. Norman J. Levy, psychiatrist, psychoanalyst, physician, member of the American Academy of Psychoanalysis, and on the staff of the Post-Graduate Center for Mental Health in New York City.

Ms. Gail Piazza, nutritionist.

Is the Lifelong Anti-Cancer Diet going to be hard to follow?

One reason that most people don't stay on a diet, even though their intentions are good when they start out, is that many diets recommend special foods that may be hard to obtain, while others are composed of dishes that are meant only for the dieter and can't be enjoyed by the entire family. Still others are expensive, or may rely on only one or two foods. And then there are the diets that leave you just plain hungry. It's no wonder that many people start a new diet every Monday, and then go off it by Friday.

But the Lifelong Anti-Cancer Diet has none of those problems. The foods on the diet are available to all, and instead of costing more money, this lifelong plan will be kind to your budget. And the person who is the cook of the household won't have to prepare food one way for the person on the plan, and another way for the rest of the family, because this plan can be followed and enjoyed by the entire family.

The diet is not meant specifically for those who want to lose weight, but you might find that as you follow this plan you will lose pounds that you had trouble shedding before.

You'll be eating foods that contain important nutrients—filling, satisfying foods that are low in calories, and won't leave you hungry—foods that can help you resist fat-rich meals that put on pounds. What a bonus— becoming healthier and slimmer at the same time! With such a possibility, shouldn't you start the Lifelong Anti-Cancer Diet today?

Am I going to feel deprived?

The feeling of deprivation is familiar to everyone who has ever gone on any diet. The advantage of the Lifelong Anti-Cancer Diet, however, is that there is no reason for you to feel hungry, although your sense of deprivation will depend on how radically different your present diet is.

If you're one of those people who subsists on coffee, diet sodas, and cigarettes one day and binges the next on cookies, potato chips, and ice cream, sure you'll feel deprived! But if you go on eating that way you'll become deprived of good health, and that's the worst loss of all.

For most people, the feeling of deprivation will be temporary, and will pass when they learn to substitute foods with important nutritional qualities for those that might be harmful to health.

The Lifelong Anti-Cancer Diet is not a rigid program that never allows a moment's deviation. It is not meant to take the joy out of life, but rather to increase the quality of life so that you will be healthier and happier.

There will be times when you won't be able to follow the plan, either because you don't want to or because you're in a situation that makes it difficult. But remember: *You can return to the plan even though you might not have followed it for one meal, or one day*. Don't allow your own personal rigidity to get in the way of good health.

It's not easy to change a way of life, a way of eating,

or a way of regarding food. Some people will examine the Lifelong Anti-Cancer Diet and find that it doesn't differ too markedly from their own way of eating, and they will have no trouble in adopting the plan and fitting it to their life-style. But you may be one of those who finds that the plan is so different from the way you currently eat that contemplating such a vast change fills you with despair. If you feel that way, try the following:

• *Ease into the plan*. For Week One choose the most appealing menus for breakfast and lunch, and eat your normal dinner. The next week, Week Two, follow the plan for breakfast, lunch, and three weekly dinners. In Week Three, try the plan for all meals. If that's too frustrating, go back to Week Two, and try again. As nutritionist Gail Piazza says, "It's a matter of reeducation—unlearning all the bad things about the way we eat, and learning all the new, good ones." Learning a new skill or art, training for a new job—all these learning procedures can be exciting. And what can be more exciting than learning to eat in a way that may save your life?

• *Don't be disappointed in yourself*. You promised yourself to follow the Lifelong Anti-Cancer Diet religiously. But this plan for good health is not a religion, and no Higher Being is going to punish you for a little backsliding. So don't punish yourself by saying, "I haven't followed the plan for the last three days, so I may as well forget the whole thing." If you haven't followed the plan one day, do your best to follow it the next. You'll soon be able to follow it every day.

• *Learn how to trade off*. Your favorite food is a hot fudge sundae with mounds of whipped cream. You've examined every page of the Lifelong Anti-Cancer Diet, and nowhere were you able to find a hot fudge sundae with whipped cream. (That's because it isn't there.) But you also feel that if you can't have a hot fudge sundae from time to time you would rather forget about the plan entirely. Life isn't worth living without a hot fudge sundae with mounds of whipped cream.

Sounds silly, doesn't it? Because in your head and your heart you know that life certainly is worth living without that hot fudge sundae. However, when you feel desperate for a certain food—and I mean really desperate—the only thing to do is to have it. Of course, this implies a controlled desperation—don't give in to that need for a hot fudge sundae too often.

Now that you've eaten that hot fudge sundae, what should you do? Don't feel guilty or anxious, because feelings of that sort are detrimental to well-being, and therefore detrimental to your health. Besides, guilt and anxiety feed upon themselves, causing more guilt and anxiety, and just might lead you to say, "I'm such a bad person that I might as well give up on the Lifelong Anti-Cancer Diet because I don't deserve to follow it."

Rather than doing that, learn to trade off. That hot fudge sundae with whipped cream was loaded with sugar and, more important, loaded with fats. For the next two or three days, avoid eating fats as much as possible. The Lifelong Anti-Cancer Diet cuts down on fats, and you can cut down even more by limiting the amount of fats used on bread or vegetables, and by cutting down the fats used in cooking.

Can I afford to follow this plan?

There are no special foods, no supplements, that you need take to enjoy the Lifelong Anti-Cancer Diet. The foods that the scientists recommend, and that are a big part of the plan, are such inexpensive and easily obtainable vegetables as carrots, sweet potatoes, cabbage, broccoli, brussels sprouts, spinach, and dried beans, and fruits such as apricots, peaches, a variety of berries, oranges, grapefruit, and raisins.

Because the committee recommended a low-fat diet you may actually find yourself spending *less* money for food, as you cut down on expensive cuts of fat-rich meats.

The report strongly suggests that important nutrients should be obtained through the foods you eat rather than through dietary supplements, so if you've been spending lots of money on bottles of mega-dose vitamins and minerals you can now apply that money to your food budget. Isn't it more enjoyable to eat a bowl of fresh, luscious red strawberries surrounded with pale-green grapefruit segments than to swallow a small yellow pill?

And when you learn how the Lifelong Anti-Cancer Diet may lessen the risk of cancer, the question becomes: "Can I afford *not* to follow the plan?"

Will I have to learn new techniques of cooking?

There are no new techniques of cooking necessary for the plan. But the report does say that *mutagens*—substances that cause mutations or inheritable changes in the genetic material of the cell—are produced when meats and fish are cooked at a very high temperature, as in charcoal broiling and in smoking. At this point, mutagens are regarded as suspect; whether they actually are carcinogens has yet to be confirmed by further testing.

"Most mutagens detected in foods have not been adequately tested for their carcinogenic activity," according to the Academy of Sciences committee. Therefore, the decision is yours as to how much food you should prepare by charcoal broiling or cooking over other high heat.

However, the committee has an additional word to

say about those mutagens: We're all eating a lot more food that has been fried in hot fat, or cooked by extreme dry heat. This includes french-fried potatoes, potato chips, fried snacks, crackers—all foods that have been highly crisped and browned.

"Many products of such browning reactions have proved to be mutagenic in laboratory tests, as have the by-products resulting from the frying and broiling of meat and fish. Hence, products in this category must be regarded as potential contributors to carcinogenesis."

The two key words here are "potential" and "carcinogenesis." Nothing has been finally proved about the mutagens, but as there is a great deal of proof associating a high-fat diet with cancer, it would seem better to have potatoes baked or mashed, to have meats and chicken potted or baked, and to have fish poached, steamed, or baked, rather than fried.

Cancer runs in my family, so if I'm going to get it anyway, why shouldn't I eat what I like?

The great good news is that many cancers are caused by environmental factors, which means that what may run in your family are dietary habits—not genetic factors—that increase the risk of cancer.

The committee offers as proof the fact that when people migrate from one country to another and adopt the dietary habits of their new country, they are also subject to the spectrum of cancers typical for that country.

It took years to correlate and gather the material for this report, because it took years to document eating patterns for groups of people, but when the information was in, the relationship of diet to cancer was so demonstrable that the report stated emphatically, "It is highly likely that the United States will eventually have the option of adopting a diet that reduces its incidence of cancer by approximately one-third.''

You could be among the one-third that are saved from cancer. Isn't that more important than following in your family's footsteps and possibly eating all the foods that could increase the risk of cancer?

Will I have to count calories on the Lifelong Anti-Cancer Diet?

The plan has not been created for people who want to lose weight.

Let's hope the plan is something you'll be able to follow easily, and for the rest of your life. There are no rigid calorie counts involved. However, the daily calorie total may be lower than that of your present diet, because of the lower fat content of the plan and because the amount of vegetables and fruits eaten at each meal will have a satisfying, filling effect, thus ending much of the yearning for high-calorie, fat-rich foods.

I've been on a high-fiber diet. Isn't this enough of a cancer preventative?

The final word is not yet in on fiber, and while the committee recommends a diet rich in fruits, vegetables, and whole grains that contain dietary fiber, it also says that various studies have both supported and contradicted the hypotheses that high-fiber diets protect against certain kinds of cancer.

While the evidence is not conclusive that fiber is protection against cancer, some laboratory studies have shown that certain types of high fiber do inhibit some colon cancers. Is it the fiber that has created this reaction, or a component of the fiber? As yet, the scientists don't know, so while you should eat foods that contain fiber, this does not mean that you don't need the Lifelong Anti-Cancer Diet as well.

Aren't I too young to worry about cancer? I'll think about that lifelong diet plan ten years from now.

Cancer can strike at any age, and the Lifelong Anti-Cancer Diet should be established as a part of your life as early as possible. It's never too soon to establish a pattern of eating that might lower the risk of cancer and that can do a great deal to help you stay healthy as you grow older.

Aren't I too old to start a new way of eating? What good can it do me now?

No one is ever too old to start on the Lifelong Anti-Cancer Diet, which might help you grow older still— far better than the other alternative. A healthy old age can be enjoyable, while an old age spent in illness can be devoid of pleasure and enjoyment.

In addition, an older person embarking on the Lifelong Anti-Cancer Diet can be an inspiration to younger members of the family, and to younger friends.

The plan limits fats. Does this include polyunsaturated fats, too?

The study explains that fats seem to increase the risk of cancer in certain areas of the body, but it also stresses limiting fats rather than excluding them. And while polyunsaturates have been cited as important in promoting the health of the heart, this report says that some laboratory studies on animals indicate that when total fat intake is low, "polyunsaturated fats are more effective than saturated fats in enhancing tumorogenesis, whereas the data on humans do not permit a clear distinction to be made between the effects of different components of fat.''

Once that's been said, what are we to do? Does this mean that we're caught between a rock and a hard place, having to choose between heart disease and cancer?

No, it doesn't mean that at all. As the report and the Lifelong Anti-Cancer Diet stress, the best plan to follow is one of moderation, which means *a diet that is low in all fats, both saturated and polyunsaturated*. The key word here is *low*, which does not mean eliminating all fats, but does mean eating *less* fat of all kinds.

Will my family like a low-fat diet?

They'll love it, because in place of the fats you'll be serving delicious dishes that will replace the unctuous quality of fat with more interesting flavors. (Our menu and recipe section will show you how.)

Many meals are prepared in such a way that they contain unnecessarily high levels of fat. You can avoid this by the following *Five Ways to Avoid Excess Fat:*

• Instead of frying or sautéeing foods, either poach, pot, braise, or steam.

• If your favorite recipe says to cook something in butter or oil, try cooking it in beef or chicken broth, or in *court bouillon* (see the recipe in Chapter Sixteen) when you're preparing fish or shellfish.

• Cut down on fat-rich meats, select lean cuts, and trim all visible fats.

• When preparing a gravy or a sauce, skim off all fat.

• Whenever possible, cut down on rich cheeses with a high butterfat content, and limit the butter or margarine you spread on bread and vegetables. Use low-fat milk and skim milk instead of whole milk some of the time.

What about my kids? They only like hot dogs, hamburgers, and french fries.

If your kids were living in Japan or in Africa they would like many other things beside hot dogs, hamburgers, and french fries. They like these foods because they're familiar; but you have to admit that they weren't born liking them.

It's up to the adults in a family to reeducate their kids, and to acquaint them with other foods besides the ones they're accustomed to. Does this mean that you can never again allow your children to have a hot dog at a baseball game or a hamburger at a barbecue? Not at all; it just means weaning them away gradually, so that their diet is varied enough to include the foods that lessen the risk of cancer.

In addition to hot dogs, hamburgers, and french fries, most of us are entirely too fond of salt-cured, preserved, and smoked foods, such as bacon, sausage, bologna, smoked ham, and smoked fish. We should eat less of them, but it's easier to learn that lesson as a child, and concerned parents can do much to start their children on a healthy diet that will benefit them throughout their lives.

Will I become thin on the Lifelong Anti-Cancer Diet?

You might, but this will depend on how closely you stick to the plan, and how *much* of the foods you eat. There is no use pretending that quantity doesn't count, and that only the quality of foods matters.

However, the plan does emphasize two important factors which should help if you're concerned about losing weight:

• The plan is low in fat, and fats are loaded with calories.

• The plan stresses the importance of vegetables and fruits, which should fill you up and lessen your hunger for weight-producing fats and sugars.

Can I follow the plan when I go to a restaurant or a party?

The plan becomes simple to follow wherever you are once you become familiar with its basic tenets, which are:

• Cut down on fats.

• Eat six or more servings per day of fruits and vegetables, with the emphasis on those fruits and vegetables rich in Vitamins A and C. A serving is ½ cup of a vegetable, and one piece of fruit.

• Eat five servings (½ cup each) a day of whole grains, which includes whole wheat bread, brown rice, corn, cornmeal, oatmeal, and barley.

• Eat two to four servings (3 to 4 ounces) each day of such protein-rich foods as fish, poultry, lean meat, eggs, and dairy products, low-fat whenever possible.

• Drink alcoholic beverages in moderation.

The Lifelong Anti-Cancer Diet was not developed with the idea of making your life more difficult; its intention is to help you avoid the risk of cancer, and to add healthy years to your life. If you regard the plan with rigidity or with grim determination, it is doubtful whether you will be able to remain on it for any worthwhile length of time.

It is not necessary to make a big speech or declaration about what you will and won't eat when you're at a restaurant or dining at a friend's house. Most restaurant menus are so varied that you should have no trouble choosing a meal that fits in perfectly with the Lifelong

Anti-Cancer Diet. An example of what you might order could be: melon or fruit cup as an appetizer; poached fish, roast veal, or a chicken dish (not fried chicken) for the main course, with salad, a baked potato, and a vegetable dish; and a fruit sorbet or a fruit tart for dessert.

Naturally, the choice is not quite that varied when you're dining at someone's home. It might be preferable to take a spoonful or two of each dish set before you—even if the dish is not part of the plan—if stating your dietary needs and requirements would make everyone at the table uncomfortable.

Besides, most people today are aware of the importance of good nutrition, and it's rare that you'll be served an entire meal of foods that might be bad for you.

If I follow the lifelong diet plan are you absolutely sure I won't come down with cancer?

There are no guarantees that this or any other plan can completely prevent all cancers. However, according to the National Academy of Sciences committee, observing dietary guidelines and recommendations can lessen the risk of cancer, especially as an estimated 30% to 40% of cancers in men and 60% of cancers in women have been attributed to a variety of environmental factors, including diet.

Cancer is not just one disease, it is actually a group of diseases, all characterized by the uncontrolled growth and spread of abnormal cells. These diseases have other environmental causes, such as smoking, overexposure to direct sunlight, and coming in contact with carcinogenic agents in the water we drink and the air we breathe, and the places where we work. Some cancers may be caused by viruses.

Obviously there are a lot of dangers we can't avoid or prevent, but if we can lessen the risk of cancer by following dietary recommendations it seems reckless and wasteful not to do so.

I've always believed that food is love, but the Lifelong Anti-Cancer Diet omits many rich goodies. How can I feed my family on a plan like that?

In recent years scientists—researchers studying heart and cancer diseases, and doctors working with them—have proved that certain foods aren't love at all. Instead they may be harmful, and can take years off someone's life. What's so loving about that?

Some foods are so associated with childhood that they symbolize love to many people. These are the soft, sweet, mushy foods of our childhood: custards, puddings, ice cream, whipped cream, muffins not merely spread with butter but lathered with it, chocolate cakes thick with icing, rice pudding enriched with many egg yolks—all the overly sweetened dishes which seemed to spell love plus rewards for a child's good behavior. These are the foods we actually have to reject now that we have become smart adults.

We know the facts—and the dangers—about a diet loaded with fat, and we also know that rich food does not mean healthful food. Scientists have demonstrated that there is a definite correlation between the diet consumed by affluent societies and the incidence of cancers of the breast, colon, and uterus.

Food can still show loving concern, especially when it incorporates the most recent scientific information and combines it with an imaginative and creative approach in menu planning and cooking. Thinking of your family's health as you cook—that's real love!

CHAPTER FOUR

HIGH-RISK FOODS: WHAT YOU SHOULD KNOW ABOUT THEM

The scientists who worked on the report issued by the National Academy of Sciences have said that no one can come up with an exact diet to protect everyone from all types of cancer—there are just too many variables, too many other factors involved. But they were able to isolate certain food categories that increase the risk of cancer at specific sites. The following is a list of those high-risk categories, and the cancers associated with them:

LIST ONE

HIGH-RISK FOOD CATEGORIES

A diet high in fats can increase the risk of cancer at the following sites:

Breast	Testes
Large bowel	Ovaries
Prostate	Gastrointestinal tract
Colon	

A diet high in very spicy foods can increase the risk of cancer at the following sites:

Stomach/gastric

A diet high in alcohol can increase the risk of cancer at the following sites:

Pancreas (limited evidence)	Liver (possible, after inducing cirrhosis)

A diet high in alcohol, combined with smoking, can increase the risk of cancer at the following sites:

Mouth	Esophagus
Larynx	Respiratory Tract

A diet high in protein can increase the risk of cancer at the following sites:

Pancreas (limited evidence)	Prostate
	Breast

A diet high in coffee can increase the risk of cancer at the following site:

Pancreas
(limited evidence)

A diet high in salt-cured, salt-pickled, and smoked foods and foods preserved with nitrates or nitrites can increase the risk of cancer at the following sites:

Esophagus	Stomach

QUESTIONS AND ANSWERS ABOUT OTHER POSSIBLE RISKS

What about a diet high in carbohydrates?

At this time there is very little known about the role of carbohydrates in the development of cancer, and while studies have suggested that a high intake of sugar might increase the risk of cancer at such sites as the pancreas and the breast, there's not enough scientific evidence to come to any definite conclusions.

What about food additives?

There are close to 3,000 substances added to the wide variety of processed foods available in the United States, plus another 12,000 chemicals involved in the materials that package these foods.

Are these additives carcinogenic? The committee reports that except for saccharin, food additives which have been tested and found to be carcinogenic in animals have been banned from use in processed foods. Thus, the use of additives does not seem to have increased the risk of cancer, but the report does say that at this time they lack adequate data to come to definite conclusions about the possibilities of such a risk.

What about artificial sweeteners?

Saccharin: Experimental studies with rats have shown that saccharin in large doses can produce tumors of the urinary tract in male rats, and can promote the action of known carcinogens in the bladders of rats. However, there has been no clear indication linking the use of nonnutritive sweeteners to cancer in humans. Most of the studies of bladder cancer have shown no association, though there have been some exceptions indicating such an association.

Aspartame: Aspartame has only recently been approved in the United States for use as an artificial sweetener, and while it's been used in Belgium and France since 1981, there are no available data as yet as to its effect on the health of human beings.

What about specific alcoholic beverages?

The report explains that alcohol and tobacco have a

definite synergistic action—that is, an action greater than merely the sum of the separate effects of alcohol and tobacco—which increases the risk for cancer of the mouth, larynx, esophagus, and respiratory tract.

But what about alcoholic beverages by themselves? At this time there are a wealth of reports indicating certain associations with cancer, but because it's hard to discover just what people mean when they say they "drink a little" or are "moderate drinkers," the panel could only suggest that alcoholic beverages be consumed in moderate amounts. What is a moderate amount? The panel of scientists didn't say, but to help you define *moderate*, consider the results of the following American and international studies. They're not conclusive, but can offer valuable guidelines.

France, 1981: In a study conducted in Lyon, patients with gastric cancer consumed about 800 calories of mostly red wine per day as compared to patients with other digestive problems who consumed 400 calories of red wine per day.

Hawaii, 1980: A direct association was observed for beer consumption and eight cancer sites: tongue/mouth, pharynx, larynx, esophagus, stomach, pancreas, lung, and kidney.

United States, 1967, 1974, 1977: Some studies demonstrated a statistically significant association between per capita beer intake and colorectal cancer, but other studies did not confirm these observations. Recently many beer manufacturers in the United States have revised the brewing process in order to reduce the amount of nitrosamines found in beer.

According to *Diet, Nutrition and Cancer* there has been some link between drinking alcoholic beverages and the development of certain cancers, but this relationship may be caused by the fact that "heavy" drinkers frequently get 25% to 50% or even more of their daily calories from alcohol. This may lead to a nutritional imbalance, which could cause a disease that might in turn lead to cancer.

MODERATION IN EVERYTHING

You now know the types of food that can increase the risk of cancer, but understand that it is impossible for most of us to use the word *never* in conjunction with food—or with anything else, for that matter. Just try a positive approach.

• Read the list of high-risk food categories (List One) again, noting as unemotionally as possible the categories that can increase the risk of cancer.

• Notice the key word in the heading over the column of food or beverage categories. The key word is *high*.

• If your daily diet contains a moderate amount of fat, or about 30% of your caloric intake, go on to the next item.

• Do you eat highly spiced foods: three times a day, once a day, once a week, or less frequently?

• Continue down the list, asking yourself honestly in which categories the word *high*, meaning large amounts, frequently consumed, applies to the foods you eat or the beverages you drink.

• Make a list of those *high* categories, and place it next to the pad you use for your shopping list, or attach it with a small magnet to your refrigerator door.

You will now have this important list before you when you plan to go marketing, or open the refrigerator door preparatory to cooking or serving a meal.

Notice that the idea here is not to say that you will never eat foods in those high categories; the only promise you need make is to cut down, to change dietary habits that could be most injurious to your health.

FOODS IN THE HIGH-RISK CATEGORIES

You now know the food categories that are associated with the possibly increased risk of cancer. There are foods in each category that most of us eat a great deal of the time. Some items may be your favorite foods, others may be unfamiliar. Understand that you may not have to cut out all these food items completely; the idea is to eat them in moderate amounts. Check the list carefully, and if some of your favorite foods appear in more than one category, plan on minimizing them in your daily diet.

For example, you'll see a number of ethnic dishes listed in the category of highly spiced foods. But just because they appear on the list doesn't mean that you can never again eat Szechuan food or have a bowl of your favorite Tex-Mex chili. The idea is to eat spicy foods in moderation, to achieve a healthy balance, and to deemphasize some of the foods that can increase the risk of cancer.

LIST TWO

THE MINUS LIST

High-Risk Category: Foods High in Fats
Dairy products:

Milk	Ice cream
Butter	Eggs

Sweet cream
Sour cream
Whole-milk yogurt
Whole-milk cheeses
(especially soft cheeses
with a high butterfat
content, such as Brie)

All oils (saturated and
polyunsaturated oils have
the same fat content)
Margarine

Meats:

Fatty cuts of beef, pork,
or lamb

Cold cuts and sausages:
bologna, frankfurters,
salami, liverwurst, pork
sausage

Miscellaneous:

Nuts
Fried foods
Mayonnaise

Non-dairy creamers
Potato chips

High-Risk Category: Foods High in Spices

Some Chinese dishes:
Szechuan and Hunanese
Some Mexican food:
dishes prepared with
hot chili peppers
"Hot" sausages
"Hot" sauces: barbecue,
Italian, East Indian, chili

Hot cherry peppers
Dishes prepared with "hot"
Hungarian paprika,
pepper flakes, Tabasco or
similar hot pepper sauce

High-Risk Category: Foods High in Protein

Beef, pork, lamb
Poultry
Cold cuts: boiled ham,
salami, turkey, corned
beef, pastrami

Fish and shellfish
Cheese
Eggs
Milk

High-Risk Category: Foods that are salt-cured, salt-pickled, smoked, prepared with nitrates or nitrites

Smoked sausages	Frankfurters
Smoked fish	Bologna
Ham	Pickled fish (herring)
Bacon	Pickled vegetables

High-Risk Category: Mutagenic foods (potential contributors to carcinogenesis if they have been crisped by exposure to heated fat, or extreme dry heat)

Fried snacks	Ready-to-eat breakfast
Crackers	cereals
	Potato chips

YOU'VE READ THE LIST . . .

You've read the list of foods in the high-risk category, and if you're like most of us who read the information for the first time, you're about to throw up your hands and decide to forget the whole thing, because too many of the foods you eat are somewhere on the list.

Don't give up, and don't despair. The panel of scientists who compiled the report are not saying that you can never, for example, eat a steak because it is high in fat and high in protein. What they are recommending is that you cut down on foods in the high-risk categories and eat more of the foods that can lessen the risk of cancer.

LEARNING TO LOOK AT FOOD IN A NEW WAY

To take full advantage of the latest scientific information linking diet to cancer you will probably have to learn to look at most foods—and at the famous four food groups—in a new way, and by doing so create different patterns of eating. For example, many of us were taught in the past that unlimited quantities of milk were good, and that no one could ever have too much protein. We're now being told that while *some* milk is good, and provides many nutrients, as does *some* protein, quantities of these foods are not the best thing for a diet that can lessen the risk of cancer.

If it just sounds like too much trouble to start rethinking old eating habits, consider the following:

• Changing the way you eat—which also means, for most of us, changing the way you cook—will give you a new interest, and the opportunity to try previously neglected foods. You'll actually be adding new flavors to your life.

• Haven't your usual daily eating patterns become just a little boring? Steak on Monday, chicken on Tuesday, the same vegetable side dishes, the same chocolate ice cream or sugar cookies for dessert? Following the Life-long Anti-Cancer Diet will give you the opportunity to experiment with foods you've probably ignored. You'll learn to prepare bulgur, whole wheat pasta, fresh fruit sorbets. The plan can become a gourmet treat!

• The high-risk category that has the longest list of foods is fats. A diet loaded with fat has long been cited as the culprit for many diseases, and too much fat makes most people gain weight, which makes them look older than they are and drains them of energy. Carrying a lot of extra weight is like carrying a lot of heavy, excess luggage, and who needs that? Cutting down on fats can be great for your looks as well as your health.

• When you recognize the importance of nutrition in relationship to cancer, and change your eating habits because of that recognition, you are actually taking charge of one aspect of your life, and becoming a more responsible, adult person. No one can regulate or predict every detail of life, but once you know there is something you can do to make your life healthier—and therefore happier—shouldn't you do it?

• The variety of foods is so great that none of us can ever hope to taste every dish, every cuisine, every fruit, vegetable, fish, or meat that is available. In view of the infinite amount of flavors in which the world abounds, it shouldn't be too hard to substitute something good for something potentially harmful.

CHAPTER FIVE

FOODS THAT CAN HELP PREVENT CANCER

The most positive aspect of the National Academy of Sciences report *Diet, Nutrition and Cancer,* on which the Lifelong Anti-Cancer Diet is based, is that there are many foods which can lessen the risk of cancer.

Best of all, they are foods that are available to all of us, and are neither rare nor expensive. You don't have to worry that the recommended foods are grown in such small quantities that only the very rich would be able to afford them, and they're not imported from faraway places that might limit the supply. These foods are so familiar, so common, that you might have been ignoring them in the mistaken belief that only the hard-to-obtain is impressive, and only rare foods can have health-giving properties.

It's time to get back to basics, and what could be more basic than the following foods recommended for your daily diet?

• *Dark-green and deep-yellow vegetables*, rich in beta-carotene, which is converted to Vitamin A in the body.

• *Cruciferous vegetables*, which means cabbage and other vegetables in that family, including broccoli, cauliflower, and brussels sprouts. Most of them contain Vitamins A and C, but the real importance of the cruciferous family is that they contain certain compounds—

isothiocyanates, indoles, and phenols—which have cancer-inhibiting effects. Enough scientific data have been accumulated to indicate that these vegetables reduce the risk of cancer at many sites.

• *Fruits,* especially citrus fruits, which are rich in Vitamin C, and other fruits rich in Vitamin A.

• *Whole grain cereals*.

LIST THREE

RISK-REDUCING FOOD CATEGORIES

A diet high in green and yellow vegetables, and other foods, such as milk, containing large quantities of Vitamin A, can reduce the risk of cancer at the following sites:

Lung	Stomach
Larynx	Colon/rectum
Bladder	Prostate
Esophagus	

A diet high in vegetables and fruits containing large quantities of Vitamin C can reduce the risk of cancer at the following sites:

Esophagus	Larynx
Stomach	Cervix/uterus (possible)

A diet high in cruciferous vegetables can reduce the risk of cancer at the following sites:

Stomach	Skin (possible)
Colon	
Rectum	

A diet high in whole grain products can reduce the risk of cancer at the following sites:

Colon (possible; evidence not yet conclusive)

Milk is listed as a source of Vitamin A, but is on the minus side for high fat. What to do?

It is true that whole milk is a great source of Vitamin A, and according to a Japanese study, daily consumption of whole milk did lower the risk for stomach cancer. However, partially skim milk is also a good source of this vitamin—and has a lower amount of fat. (Completely skim milk, which is fine in the low-fat area, has only a very small amount of Vitamin A.)

The answer is not to expect to get your entire daily quota of Vitamin A from milk. Vegetables such as carrots and broccoli also contain a great deal of Vitamin A, as do fruits such as apricots and avocados (yes, avocado is a fruit). You can combine a number of sources to obtain a sufficient amount of Vitamin A.

You list whole grain products but you don't mention fiber. Why?

The final word is not yet in on fiber, though the report from the National Academy of Sciences does mention a number of studies indicating that fiber may have some protective effect against both colon and rectal cancer.

Scientists are continuing to analyze the individual properties of fiber, and there seems to be enough positive evidence for a recommendation of whole grain products which do contain fiber.

In addition to fiber, however, whole grain products also contain Vitamin E, and this vitamin has been shown to inhibit the formation of *nitrosamines*—highly carcinogenic chemicals.

I've tried to follow a high-protein diet for years, because it's one way I found to keep my weight down. What should I do now?

Much high-protein food is also high-fat, and fat, according to the study, is one food component that increases the risk for many cancers. However, *cutting down* on fatty foods does not mean that you have to *cut out* protein—just reduce your intake, and whenever possible, choose protein-rich foods that are lower in fats, such as poultry, fish, eggs, beans, and lean meat as opposed to high-fat meats.

Americans, as a rule, do eat a diet high in protein, and because most of it is animal protein, it's hard to separate the effects of fat from the effects of protein.

You can still have two to four servings of protein-rich foods each day. The idea is not to have mainly protein, excluding other important foods. And, by the way, soybean products are loaded with protein, as well as with compounds called *protease inhibitors*, which have been shown to reduce the incidence of certain cancers in laboratory animals. If soybean doesn't charm you as much as a rare steak, just try to remember that the Japanese call soybean curd *tofu*—"meat without bones."

I don't mind eating raw carrot sticks, or raw cabbage in cole slaw, but I hate those vegetables cooked. Is it just as good to eat them raw?

Some of the studies citing the effectiveness of certain vegetables said that they had been eaten raw, and nutritionists for years have been advising people not to cook vegetables to death. Do eat carrots and cabbage raw, and see the recipe section of this book for a low-fat dip, to serve with carrot sticks, and a different dressing for cole slaw.

How can I cook vegetables to best preserve vitamins and other nutrients?

When cooking vegetables, less is definitely better in every way: Use less liquid, and less time. The longer you cook vegetables the more nutrients will be destroyed.

Steam vegetables, or stir-fry them quickly. If you wish, cook them in a small amount of boiling water, and save the water to add to sauces or soups.

Whenever possible, use pots or pans that have a nonstick surface so that you can eliminate cooking oils or fats.

If possible, try to cook just as much as you need for each day. Leftover vegetables that have been cooked and stored in the refrigerator for a few days lose much of their Vitamin C when they are reheated.

Wash vegetables before you cook them, but wash them as quickly as you can; do not keep them soaking in water. Water can wash off the surface vitamins and minerals.

Are you advocating a vegetarian diet? Is that what the Lifelong Anti-Cancer Diet is going to be?

Not at all. The Lifelong Anti-Cancer Diet is not a vegetarian diet, though with a few adjustments vegetarians will be able to follow it quite easily. It is a plan that takes advantage of the latest scientific findings that indicate the relationship between diet and cancer, and therefore places emphasis on foods that can lower the risk of cancer—mostly fruits, vegetables, and whole grains.

But meat, poultry, and fish all have their place in the plan, as do other foods.

Why don't we just cut out all the foods on the minus list?

Some of the foods on the Minus List (List Two) should not be cut out entirely. Many foods high in fats, for example, provide needed calcium, while foods high in protein are necessary for building new body tissue and for producing enzymes necessary for normal body functions. Still other foods on the Minus List contain important vitamins and minerals necessary to all-round good health.

However, if you wish to eliminate spicy, pickled, smoked, and salt-cured foods and alcohol entirely from your diet, you may do so without creating any nutritional imbalance.

You mention foods that are rich in Vitamins A and C. Aren't the other vitamins important, too?

Other vitamins and minerals are also important and should be part of everyone's daily diet. The reason the Lifelong Anti-Cancer Diet emphasizes Vitamins A and C is that these are the vitamins that have been shown to reduce the risk of cancer.

FOODS THAT MAY REDUCE THE RISK OF CANCER

The Plus List indicates the categories that can reduce the risk of cancer, and there is a selected source of items in each category. Read the list carefully, and then read it once again. Use it as a guide for menu planning and marketing. Many of the items should be staples of your daily diet.

LIST FOUR

PLUS LIST

Risk-Reducing Category: Foods High in Vitamin A

Vegetables:

Broccoli

Carrots

Chinese cabbage
  (bok choy)

Lettuce: escarole,
  romaine, bibb

Kale

Mustard greens

Peas

Sweet red peppers

Pumpkin

Spinach

Winter squash

Sweet potatoes (not the
  same as yams)

Swiss chard

Fruits:

Apricots

Avocado

Cantaloupe

Grapefruit

Mangos

Nectarines

Peaches

Persimmons

Dairy products (low-fat when possible)

Milk

Ricotta cheese

Cheddar cheese

Fish and shellfish:

Crab

Halibut

Lobster

Mackerel

Salmon

Swordfish

Meats:

Liver

Kidneys

Risk-Reducing Category: Foods High in Vitamin C

Vegetables:

Broccoli	Mustard greens
Brussels sprouts	Green peppers
Cauliflower	Red peppers
Celery	Tomatoes
Kale	

Fruits:

Cantaloupe	Mangos
Currants	Oranges
Grapefruit	Papaya
Kiwi fruit	Strawberries

Risk-Reducing Category: Cruciferous vegetables

Cabbage	Cauliflower
Broccoli	Kale
Brussels sprouts	

Risk-Reducing Category: Whole grain products

Whole wheat bread	Barley
Oatmeal	Buckwheat groats
Brown rice	Bulgur
Wheat germ	Corn
Bran	Cornmeal

THE CROSS OVER AND CROSS OUT SHOPPING LIST

You have now read the important Four Lists:

• *List One*: Food categories that could increase the risk of cancer.

• *List Two*: The Minus List of foods that should be minimized in your diet.

• *List Three*: Food categories that can help reduce the risk of cancer.

• *List Four*: The Plus List of foods that should be emphasized in your daily diet.

Making Out a Shopping List

Before consulting the Four Lists, make out your own regular shopping list. Write down the foods that you would normally buy if you hadn't read any part of this book.

Now, your list in hand, compare it to the Four Lists. How many of the foods on your list are on the minus list? Just a few? Many? Practically all? Perhaps you never realized just how great an emphasis you were placing on foods that could be potentially dangerous if eaten in large amounts, and eaten without thought of the foods on the Plus List.

If the meals you've been eating are mainly hamburgers, frankfurters, and french fries, or if you've been eating large quantities of fried foods and ice cream, with just an occasional salad thrown in for color, consider changing your dietary habits today—right now—with the shopping list you're presently holding in your hand. Just remember that this is the first day of the rest of your life, and you want the rest of your life to be as healthy as possible!

Crossing Out

Throw out your old shopping list—or, if you wish, cross out as many of the unnecessary high-risk items as possible (you won't be able to cross them all out; some should be eaten in moderation, and you might not be able to part from other favorites the first time out). Now, start all over again.

Make a new list based on as many of the Plus List foods as possible, and cut down on the Minus List foods wherever you think you can. Build your main courses around vegetables and your desserts around fruits, and be sure to include whole grain items.

Remember, what we're planning here is not a crash diet, or a one-food diet, or a fad diet that is unpleasantly limiting. If anything, the Lifelong Anti-Cancer Diet should expand your food horizons, just as it might expand your life.

Crossing Over

It is hard to change what may have been eating habits of a lifetime, but it can be done. You can cross over from the Minus List to the Plus List. Here are some suggestions as to how you can do it a step at a time:

• Have your breakfasts been mainly eggs with bacon or ham?

CROSS OVER TO: Half a grapefruit or a slice of cantaloupe, followed by a corn muffin, or a whole wheat blueberry muffin with strawberry preserves.

• Is your preferred lunch a hamburger with french fries?

CROSS OVER TO: A glass of tomato juice with a wedge of lemon, followed by a spinach salad, and a whole wheat roll with 1 pat of butter or margarine. For dessert have a nectarine, peach, or banana.

- For dinner do you often have a large slice of roast beef with a baked potato dripping with butter, a small salad, and a piece of cake or ice cream?

    CROSS OVER TO: Pasta with a sauce of chopped fresh tomatoes, basil, garlic, and a small amount of olive oil, followed by roast chicken with herbed brown rice, and a cassis or melon sorbet.

These are only a few suggested ways in which you can change your eating habits. You'll find a larger group of menus as well as recipes later on in this book. However, to accomplish this *crossover* you must be prepared to *cross out* some of the familiar items on your shopping list. To do so, consider the following:

- *Change your pattern of marketing.*

Most of us enter a supermarket and start down the same aisle each time we walk into the store. The store has become familiar, as are the foods we choose to eat.

Now is the time for a change! Approach the food store as though you've never been there before. If you usually walk down the right or left aisle first, walk down the center aisle this time.

Just walking through a store in a new direction will enable you to see items that you may never have noticed before, and they may help you create a new pattern of eating.

- *Go to the meat counter last.*

Many people, unless they follow a vegetarian diet, head for the meat counter first, and build their meals around a meat main dish.

Instead of doing that, go to the vegetable and fruit section first. Plan a main entree around vegetables. This doesn't mean that you should completely eliminate meats from your food plan, it just means that meats need not be the centerpiece, but should provide an interesting fillip of taste and texture to complement important vegetables.

• *Consider fresh fruits for dessert.*

Walk on past the frozen-food case holding that array of ice cream, and concentrate on fresh fruits, instead. Fruit does not have to be eaten plain and uncooked every time. How about poached peaches in wine, or apricot whip, or a compote of fruits? If you can't live without something creamy, try an ice milk with a lower fat content, or spoon the compote of fruits over well-chilled low-fat yogurt.

• *Search out the unusual.*

Have you ever tried whole wheat pasta? Sun-dried tomatoes? Wheat-flour burritos? Whole wheat pita bread? These and other new and interesting food items are waiting for you at most food stores. Just because certain foods are healthier than others does not mean that they have to be dull or limited in flavors.

• *A snack does not always have to be chips, pretzels, or crackers and cheese.*

It can be fresh vegetables: a platter of carrot sticks, celery hearts, cauliflower sprigs, and sugar snap peas surrounding a low-fat dip; the colors are beautiful, the tastes are varied, the textures offer a satisfying crunch, and you'll be eating something low in fats, and high in wonderful nutrients, and eliminating crackers, pretzels, and chips, which have been cooked either in hot fat or in dry high heat.

Or try pureed chick peas mixed with a sesame-seed spread, and offered with triangles of whole wheat pita bread—another snack that's delicious and provides protein and important whole grains.

Little by little, as you become more familiar with the

Lifelong Anti-Cancer Diet, you will find it easier to *cross out* food items that lack nutritional qualities, and you will have *crossed over* to a healthier way of eating.

CHAPTER SIX

VITAMINS AND MINERALS

Too many of us tend to skip a meal and take a pill; or go on a crash diet (must-lose-20-pounds-before-I-go-on-vacation) and take another pill. And now that the report of the National Academy of Sciences has been issued, placing special emphasis on the benefits of Vitamins A and C, some of us may dash out to our neighborhood pharmacy or health-food store to purchase still another bottle of megadose vitamins and minerals.

Unless you have consulted with your doctor and he or she has given you some special reasons why you should take dietary supplements—don't do it!

According to the panel of scientists who worked on the report, ". . . there is very little information on the effects of various levels of individual nutrients on the risk of cancer in humans. Therefore, the committee is unable to predict the health effects of high and potentially toxic doses of isolated nutrients consumed in the form of supplements."

But, you're asking, if there are certain vitamins that can lower the risk of cancer—and there seem to be—why not take a handful of the little pills that contain megadoses of those vitamins?

The answer is that while a proper amount of vitamins and minerals can promote health, an overdose could be harmful, and no pill can take the place of the type of balanced diet recommended by the Lifelong Anti-Cancer Diet.

Do you remember how you felt the last time you went on a crash diet for a number of days? Or the time you were too busy to eat properly? Didn't you feel irritable, and slightly sick without knowing exactly why you felt that way? No amount of dietary supplements can rid you of those quirky sensations, but a proper diet can relieve the sick symptoms caused by inadequate meals.

The importance of Vitamins A and C has been discussed in previous chapters, but if you want further documented proof as well as information about other vitamins and minerals, here it is:

VITAMINS

What can Vitamin A do for you? In quite a number of studies conducted in the United States, Iran, Japan, and England it was discovered that Vitamin A lowered the risk of cancer of the lung, larynx, bladder, esophagus, stomach, colon/rectum, and prostate.

What happens if you have a Vitamin A Deficiency? Some studies have shown that a deficiency of Vitamin A can result in a greater susceptibility of the body to cancerous growths.

What happens if you take too much Vitamin A? Too much Vitamin A can be toxic, and can cause anorexia (loss of appetite), loss of hair, drying of skin, bone fragility, and enlargement of the liver and the spleen.

What can Vitamin C do for you? The results of studies indicated that foods rich in Vitamin C lowered the risk of cancers of the stomach and the esophagus.

What happens if you have a Vitamin C Deficiency? In

addition to the possibility that you will be more susceptible to certain cancers—and according to some scientists to more colds—a lack of Vitamin C also retards the
healing of wounds and causes swelling and infection of
the gums and pains of the joints.

What happens if you take too much Vitamin C? Vitamin C is not retained in the system as is Vitamin A, but
there have been some associations of urinary-tract problems with megadoses of Vitamin C.

What can Vitamin E do for you? Vitamin E is present
in so many foods—eggs, vegetable oils, and whole
grain cereal products—that it's hard to identify the exact
amount of Vitamin E that most people receive from
their diet. At this time, the studies done on Vitamin E
are incomplete, but laboratory tests done *in vivo* and *in
vitro*—which means tests done with animals and in test
tubes—have indicated that Vitamin E does inhibit the
formation of nitrosamines, which are carcinogenic
chemicals.

What happens if you have a Vitamin E Deficiency?
Vitamin E works as an antioxidant, and by accepting
oxygen it works to preserve the important Vitamin A in
the body. Other plus factors have been attributed to this
vitamin, but though we know Vitamin E is necessary,
its complete significance is not yet clear.

What happens if you take too much Vitamin E? At
this time, there's not enough information regarding the
toxic level of Vitamin E, but as so many foods contain
Vitamin E, why take a pill?

*What can Vitamin B Complex and choline do for
you?* The B Vitamins have not been studied sufficiently
to indicate a relationship between these vitamins and
cancer, but nutritionists agree that this spectrum of vitamins is necessary to good health.

Because this book deals specifically with the effects

of diet on cancer as documented by the National Academy of Sciences report, there won't be a discussion here of all the other essential vitamins. If you want to know whether or not you should take daily supplements, you should discuss the question with your doctor.

MINERALS

The panel of scientists made no further report on other vitamins, but they did offer information on nine minerals both nutritive and nonnutritive, and their relation to cancer.

Nutritive Minerals

Selenium: Selenium has been studied to discover its relationship to cancer, both as a causative and as a preventative agent. During the past forty years it has been described as both a carcinogen and an anticarcinogen, based on animal studies. Some selenium may be good, but too much selenium can be dangerous.

What you can do about selenium: Increasing the dosage of selenium by supplements has not been shown to confer health benefits, say the scientists, and the recommendation is to rely on the selenium available in a balanced diet. Selenium is derived from water, and from foods grown on soil that contains this mineral.

Zinc: When studies were made regarding zinc in diet the results were contradictory. Experiments in animals have shown that zinc can either enhance or retard tumor growth. Zinc is important to a healthily functioning body, and can be obtained from many food sources.

What you can do about zinc: Zinc is found in meat,

liver, eggs, poultry, and seafood. Oysters are especially rich in zinc. Milk, whole grain products, and yeast are also sources of zinc. According to *Medical Letter*, a pharmaceutical advisory bulletin for doctors, "There is no evidence that zinc supplements offer any benefit for healthy people, and they may be hazardous."

Iron: Iron deficiency has been associated with an increased risk of cancer of the upper alimentary tract, including the stomach and the esophagus. Exposure to iron by inhalation can increase the risk of cancer, while high levels of iron in the diet do not.

What you can do about iron: Eat foods rich in iron. Among them are liver, spinach and other dark-green vegetables, dried beans, dried fruits, raisins, and meat.

Copper: Copper is an essential nutrient, but studies relating cancer to dietary copper are inconclusive. Copper may be carcinogenic, but dietary sources of copper have not so far been implicated.

What you can do about copper: Copper is widely distributed in foods, and may be in drinking water. Copper helps the body absorb iron, and also works to metabolize Vitamin C. You can receive a sufficient amount of copper if you include liver, shellfish, meats, nuts, dried beans, and whole grain cereals in your diet.

Iodine: There is some evidence, though limited, that an iodine deficiency can increase the risk of thyroid cancer in humans. Some studies have indicated that excessive iodine may increase the risk of thyroid cancer, but these studies have not been confirmed, and studies with animals support the association between iodine deficiency and cancer.

What you can do about iodine: Use iodized salt, and eat shrimp, oysters, mussels, scallops, crab, lobster, and saltwater fish. Fluoridated water also contains iodine.

Molybdenum: There have been very few studies done

regarding the link between molybdenum deficiency and cancer.

The most interesting study is being conducted in China. Molybdenum has been added to molybdenum-poor soil in an area where the rate for esophageal cancer is high. The molybdenum has increased the ascorbic acid content of the soil, and decreased the nitrates and nitrites. These changes are reflected in the plant life, and now the results of this scientific mystery story are awaited: Will plants with a lower nitrate and nitrite context lower the incidence of esophageal cancer?

Elsewhere only one study has so far indicated that molybdenum might have an effect on tumors of the esophagus and the forestomach caused by nitrosamines.

What you can do about molybdenum: Molybdenum is a trace element, meaning that it appears only in traces, and only minute quantities of it are needed. Molybdenum is obtained from dried beans, whole grain cereals, and organ meats.

Nonnutritive Minerals

Cadmium: Cadmium may be one of the trace elements in the water supply. Smoking cigarettes and engaging in certain occupations also increase exposure to cadmium. Some studies indicate that dietary exposure to cadmium is associated with an increased risk of cancer, but other studies don't confirm this, and therefore the scientific panel has not come to any definite conclusions about the relation of dietary cadmium to cancer.

Arsenic: Arsenic is one of the trace elements in the soils and waters of the world. It can be present in such foods as fruits and potatoes where an insecticide containing an arsenic derivative is used. A low level of arsenic may also be present in dairy products, and in meat, fish, and poultry.

If drinking water is heavily contaminated with arsenic it can increase the risk of skin cancer. However, because animals, unlike humans, are not susceptible to arsenic-induced cancer, there aren't sufficient data to say whether or not normally low levels of arsenic in the diet increase the risk of cancer.

Lead: We are exposed to lead through such environmental sources as automobile exhausts, atmospheric dust, drinking water, food, and paint. Lead in drinking water has been directly related to the increase of cancer of the stomach, small intestine, large intestine, ovary, and kidney, as well as myeloma, lymphomas, and leukemia. Lead in food—as in the residue left after fruit has been sprayed with lead arsenate—has not been linked to cancer.

CHAPTER SEVEN

THE WORD IS NOT YET IN ON . . .

Have you read that coffee may increase the risk of cancer? That overweight is a factor? What about cholesterol? Here is the latest information on these and other dietary components.

High-calorie diet: Obesity has been linked to many health problems, including heart disease. But what relationship—if any—do too many calories and overweight have to cancer?

At this point it's hard to say. Scientists are having difficulty distinguishing between total caloric intake versus total fat and protein intake in regard to cancer.

Some studies suggest that weight could influence the risk of breast cancer, but the results are inconclusive. Trying to pinpoint cause to effect results in some mazelike thinking:

(1) Obese people do take in more calories than necessary; (2) some of those calories may come from fat, and fat does increase the risk of cancer; therefore (3), is it fat or fat plus overweight that is the villain?

At this point, the panel of scientists believe that fat intake rather than overweight is more relevant, but they also add that laboratory studies indicate that a diet lower in calories does decrease the chances of cancer in animals.

Is the same true for humans? At this time the evidence for humans is less clear.

Cholesterol: This is another one of those scientific mysteries. High cholesterol is associated with heart disease, and some studies have indicated a correlation between a high fat/high cholesterol diet and cancer of the colon.

However, other studies have shown the opposite, and some cancer patients in a number of studies have had low levels of serum cholesterol. One wonders which came first, the low level of serum cholesterol or the cancer.

At this time the data are inconsistent. An inverse correlation between serum cholesterol and colon cancer in men has been noted in some studies, but not in all. And other data have indicated lower cholesterol levels in cancer patients. The report says that ''low serum cholesterol levels may be a clue to some unknown factor.''

Scientists will continue to study the effects of high or low cholesterol on cancer incidence.

Carbohydrates (sugars and starches): Scientists agree that carbohydrates require more research. One study related cancer of the pancreas in women to sugar; another linked a high intake of refined sugar combined with a low intake of starch to an increased incidence of breast cancer. But two other studies associated a high intake of starch with a high incidence of gastric and esophageal cancer.

The evidence, say the scientists, is still too meager for them to say that sugars and starches play a part in cancer incidence. But they do say that too many carbohydrates could mean too many calories, and an excess of calories may have something to do with cancer incidence.

Coffee: Here are the pros and cons of the Coffee Question.

1. Some case studies have linked coffee drinking with an elevated risk for cancer of the bladder.
2. Other studies have not confirmed this, and in laboratory tests, there were no tumors of the bladder noted in animals that were fed a diet high in coffee.
3. A number of studies have made an association between the consumption of both regular coffee and decaffeinated coffee with cancer of the pancreas.
4. In studies with animals, it was found that high levels of caffeine led to a lower incidence of tumors.
5. Some studies have associated coffee consumption with renal and prostate cancer, but other studies have not confirmed these findings.
6. One study which analyzed the chemical compounds which go to make up coffee indicated that one component (not caffeine) did act as a catalyst in the formation of nitrosamines—carcinogenic chemicals. Says the report, "This finding implies that several foodstuffs and beverages, including coffee, may have cocarcinogenic properties." (A *cocarcinogen* is a substance that in combination with a carcinogen can increase the risk of cancer.)

Protein: A number of studies have suggested a possible link between high levels of protein and an increased risk of cancer of the breast, pancreas, kidney, prostate, and endometrium.

However, because most of the high-protein foods we eat are also high in fat, and because a high-fat diet has been associated with cancer, fat could be the more important element in a link with cancer.

But, says the panel of scientists, "the evidence does not completely preclude an independent effect of protein.'' The evidence suggests that protein intake just *may* increase the risk of cancer, but until more studies are done, separating the effects of fat from the effects of protein, the scientists have not been able to come to any ''firm conclusion about the independent effect of protein.''

Nitrates and Nitrites: Nitrates and nitrites are used as preservatives for curing meats and for preserving other products. Bacon, frankfurters, salami, and other cured meats as well as some baked goods and cereals are among the foods that may contain these preservatives.

Some studies have indicated that a higher rate of cancers of the stomach and the esophagus is linked with a high level of nitrate or nitrite in the diet or the drinking water.

Nitrite, while not a cancer-causing agent by itself, could interact with other dietary components to produce a compound that might induce cancer.

The evidence about nitrates, nitrites, and their derivative, *N*-nitroso compounds, are inconclusive. However, high levels of nitrates and nitrites have been associated with an increased incidence of cancers of the stomach and the esophagus.

Diet, Nutrition and Cancer reported the findings of an earlier committee of scientists which recommended that ''exposure to nitrate, nitrite and *N*-nitroso compounds should be reduced.''

HOW MUCH SHOULD YOU CHANGE YOUR WAY OF LIFE?

You've now read the latest findings on high-calorie diets, cholesterol, carbohydrates, coffee, protein, and nitrates and nitrites.

The findings are inconclusive, but some of the above

categories could increase the risk of cancer. Notice that in most cases, the scientists used the word *high* and *excess* when describing the possible relation of these elements to cancer.

At this time no one is saying that you may never have another cup of coffee, another steak or potato, or another slice of ham or bacon.

What is suggested is moderation. Possibilities of danger lurk in overdoing, in eating foods in certain categories to excess. Instead of feeling defeated by the very idea of having to *cut out* many of your favorite foods or beverages, consider *cutting down*.

CHAPTER EIGHT

A LIFE-AFFIRMING PHILOSOPHY

Why do we eat foods we know are bad for us?

Why do we do things that are damaging to our health?

These are some of the questions I asked Dr. Norman J. Levy, psychiatrist, psychoanalyst, and physician. We discussed some of the reasons—conscious and subconscious—that people have for acting out self-destructive impulses. According to Dr. Levy, we all need a life-affirming philosophy, and acquiring such a philosophy takes both insight and a healthy amount of self-interest.

I don't mean to eat all the wrong foods, but sometimes I just can't help it. Or can I?

You have to like yourself enough to do the best for yourself. Sure, certain things may taste good, but if they're not in your best interests you have to cut down, or exclude them. That's in the interest of being in good health, of staying alive.

Do I have to follow a rigid diet?

Rigid diets don't work. If you intend to stay on a diet forever, it can't be rigid, or you won't stay on it. And some rigid diets turn out to be bad for you. It was recently discovered that people who cut out fats entirely— who never had butter, or cream, or cheese—reduced the calcium in their systems to such a degree that the result was high blood pressure.

I look at certain foods, like a candy bar, as a reward. Why is that?

Either you believe that you've done something special, something good, and you feel you can reward yourself with a treat—a childish treat, if it's a candy bar—or you're anxious, and you're eating that candy bar to fill an inner emptiness.

Can I learn to find more substantial rewards? A candy bar isn't really very much.

Food is a substitute for a real reward, and eating is not the answer to anxiety. Try to understand what is going on within. Learn more about yourself, and about the motives that drive you into the state that makes you reach out for too much food, or food that isn't good for you.

Life is so frustrating—why should I frustrate myself about food?

You'll feel more frustrated if you can't walk away from something that is bad for you—something injurious to your health. Imagine your frustration when you have to admit that you have no control over yourself.

I think I'm on the right path. I jog and play tennis. Isn't that good?

That's great. You like yourself enough to take care of your body. Now learn to care still more by following dietary guidelines.

I'm on the verge of divorce. And if that isn't bad enough, I feel hungry all the time. Why is that?

If you're involved in a bad relationship, a relationship in which you feel ignored or unloved, you're probably also in a state of rage. Perhaps the only way you can keep that rage in control is by eating—by filling an emotional emptiness with food you really don't need, and actually don't want. As you work out the problems in your relationship, and your resentment and rage lessen, your appetite will probably lessen, too.

I know I eat a lot of the wrong foods. But I just can't get myself to care about what I eat. I don't believe it will make a difference.

For some reason, you're feeling hopeless about your life, and your attitude about eating wrong foods is just another manifestation of your down mood. But this can be a vicious circle. You know you're doing something wrong—something bad for your health—and you punish yourself still further by continuing to do the wrong thing that made you dislike yourself in the first place.

Try to understand the emotions that are driving you into a potentially destructive situation. You need relief from the pressures that push you in that direction, so that you can fulfill yourself instead of destroying yourself.

If I can never eat a plate of french fries again, I think I'd just as soon forget the whole diet.

Just think of the diet one day at a time. Don't make any absolute rules. Don't say "I will never, ever eat a french fry, not for the rest of my life." Just say "I won't eat a french fry today."

If you think of not eating something ever again, it's pretty terrible, but twenty-four hours—that isn't so bad.

I've tried other diets, but I can never stay on them. Will this diet be easier to follow?

Maybe you look at diets with too much rigidity. If you do go off the diet every so often, try not to get too anxious. Anxiety can do more harm than anything, and it can drive you to do all the wrong things. If you stray from the diet for a day or two, try to cut down during the next few days on the foods you've been overindulging in—the foods you know are not good for you.

I just don't believe that cancer can happen to me. Why should I follow the diet?

That sounds like arrogance. You have arrogated to yourself the power to transcend the normal. Perhaps in time you will come to understand that you just don't have that power.

Possibly it isn't arrogance, but an unconscious desire to harm yourself. It's important to understand your real motives, your real reasons for doing something against your own best self-interests.

I'm definitely going on the Lifetime Anti-Cancer Diet. Should I make my family go along with me?

Don't make your family's life miserable by being so overanxious that you can't allow yourself and your family the freedom of a "sometimes" or an "occasionally." If you try to have complete control over every morsel your family eats you might drive them to do just the opposite—to eat all the things that they know are bad for them—not in defiance of the foods, but in defiance of the way you lay down the rules. Ease into the diet without too much discussion.

I had an uncle who smoked, and ate all those high-risk foods, and he lived to be ninety. Are you going to give me a guarantee to go along with the diet?

There are no guarantees, of course. But there are no guarantees that you'll have your uncle's kind of good luck, either.

I'm not an important person. Who cares about what happens to me?

You have to care. You have to like yourself enough to do what is best for yourself. You have a place on earth, as does everyone, and you can make a contribution, even though it isn't earth-shaking. Besides, you are an important person to your family and friends, and you can contribute to their emotional well-being by staying healthy—staying alive.

CHAPTER NINE

NEW WAYS OF LOOKING AT FOODS

How can you best handle your decision to change the way you eat? Try the following:

1. *Make no rigid resolutions*. Don't say to yourself— or to anyone else—that from tomorrow on you will never again eat well-marbled meat or a hot dog at the ball park.

2. *Face up to your own reluctance* to live by an either-or decision. Try to think, act, and feel more moderately about changing your style of eating.

3. *Cut down* on foods that carry an element of risk, but cut down gradually.

4. *Send in the substitutes*. For example, you now know that it isn't the caffeine in coffee that increases the risk of cancer, and therefore that decaffeinated coffee is not an anti-cancer substitute for regular coffee. (If caffeine causes other problems, then consider decaffeinated coffee for those reasons.)

However, there are other beverages that contain the caffeine that your system, or personality, may require, so instead of drinking unlimited amounts of coffee, alternate with tea, or other drinks with caffeine.

Want to cut down on cholesterol, protein, and nitrates and nitrites all at the same time? Cut down on favorite delicatessen items—ham, pastrami, corned beef, frankfurters. If you want meat for a sandwich, how about slices of roast breast of turkey, instead?

Use substitutes some of the time for foods that contain an element of risk.

5. *Analyze your cravings.* For example, just why do you feel you must have that rich dessert which you know is loaded with fat, calories, and cholesterol? Ask yourself if you're eating that dessert because:
   a. It's a habit.
   b. You need it.
   c. You don't believe the report, and besides, cancer won't strike you.

ANALYZING THE REASONS

If you checked "a," and you're eating that dessert as a matter of habit, understand that you weren't born with a sweet tooth, or a fat tooth. Habits can be changed, and a capacity to change indicates an open mind, a greater interest in life, and a willingness to examine new evidence as it comes along. Change your habit of eating rich desserts— not all of the time, just most of the time.

If you checked "b," why do you need that dessert? If you're still hungry, have more of the main course or the salad, or have another slice of bread (not white bread, if possible). If it's too late to do that, remember the next time to fill up before dessert comes around.

If you're substituting that rich dessert for other rewards, admit to yourself that food can't take the place of love, recognition, or money. Eating too many rich desserts will make you feel inadequate about your own capacity to control your life, and if you don't feel good about yourself, it will be even harder to go after the real rewards you should have.

The report is so well documented that lack of curiosity about it indicates the mind of an ostrich—not the prettiest or smartest of birds. If you checked "c," pick your head up out of the sand, open your eyes, and take another look at the scientific facts and figures. It may not be convenient to believe the report, but not believing it won't make it go away, or be less true. Does hedonism stand in the way, by chance?

Cancer can strike anyone, and by eating badly you add to the risk. Why use diet as a game of Russian roulette? Take up sky diving, instead.

6. *Assess your own capacity for change.* How often are you willing to change the styles and patterns of your daily life? Are you open to new people, new ideas? Do you ever change the way you walk or drive to work, the length of your skirts, or the width of your neckties? If not, you may be getting into a rut. Consider change as a constructive element rather than a measure to be feared, and understand that changing the way you eat can be one of the most beneficial acts of your life.

7. *Look at it as a worthwhile trade.* There is a possibility that you might lessen the risk of cancer if you give up some—not all—bad eating habits.

8. *Look forward, not back.* Don't worry about past indulgences. The past can't be changed, but the future can!

9. *Think of all the people who care for you*—your family and friends.

10. *Be good to yourself,* and cut down on food risks when possible. You deserve good health!

CHAPTER TEN

THE LIFELONG ANTI-CANCER DIET IN DETAIL—THE 21-DAY MENU PLAN

Earlier in this book you read the new, exciting, and hope-inspiring information based on the National Academy of Sciences report linking diet to cancer. You now know that what you eat might increase or reduce the risk of cancer, and as the report states, "It is highly likely that the United States will eventually have the option of adopting a diet that reduces its incidence of cancer by one-third."

The report made specific recommendations and offered dietary guidelines. How can you apply these recommendations and guidelines to your life, and the lives of those you love?

This is where the Lifelong Anti-Cancer Diet comes in. The diet follows the guideline with a 21-Day Menu Plan (plus a week of optional menus for variety) which illustrates how you can make this new body of scientific information part of your daily life.

The plan places particular emphasis on the Big Basics of the report, which are:

SEVEN BIG BASICS OF LESS AND MORE

MORE   LESS

Eat more: Eat less:

1. Foods rich in   1. Fats
   Vitamin A   2. Protein foods that are
2. Foods rich in   especially rich in fats
   Vitamin C   3. Salt-cured, salt-pickled,
3. Cruciferous vegetables   and smoked foods
4. Whole grain foods

In addition to the Seven Big Basics, there are other important recommendations to keep in mind, and these are:

1. Cut down on foods cooked in heated fat or over extreme dry heat, such as:
   • Fried foods
   • Crispy and brown crackers and snacks
   • Potato chips
   • Ready-to-eat breakfast cereals
2. Unless your doctor tells you to do otherwise, plan on getting your full complement of vitamins and minerals from the foods you eat rather than from dietary supplements.
3. Drink in moderation, and remember that alcohol may combine with inhaled cigarette smoke to increase the risk of certain cancers.

THE LIFELONG ANTI-CANCER DIET PLAN CHART

The following chart indicates foods, by category, to be included in your daily diet.

Remember that if for any one of a number of reasons— you may be traveling, visiting, too busy to eat—there is a day when you just can't follow the recommendations on the chart, all is not lost. This is a *lifelong* diet plan, and there are unpredictable events in everyone's life that necessitate adjustments.

Don't let one bad day make you abandon the Lifelong Anti-Cancer Diet forever. Return to it as soon as you can. You'll find, in time, that following the diet becomes easier and easier. Food preferences can change, and soon your tastes will come to reflect the dietary guidelines suggested by the National Academy of Sciences report.

FOODS TO BE INCLUDED IN DAILY DIET

FRUITS, VEGETABLES		*WHOLE GRAINS, CEREALS*	*PROTEIN*
*6 or More Servings**		*5 Servings**	*2–4 Servings**
Fruits and vegetables rich in Vitamins A and C, and cruciferous vegetables:		Whole grain products:	Meats, fish, poultry, eggs
		Whole wheat breads	Legumes: dried beans,
Apricots	Broccoli	Brown rice	chickpeas,
Citrus fruits	Brussels	Barley	dried peas,
Cantaloupe	Sprouts	Wheat germ	lentils, soy-
Cherries	Cabbage	Bulgur	beans, tofu
Kiwi fruit	Carrots	Bran	
Mango	Cauliflower	Oatmeal	
Pap_a	Escarole	Buckwheat	Dairy products:
Peaches	Kale	groats,	milk,
Watermelon	Parsley	(kasha)	cheese,

FRUITS, VEGETABLES	*WHOLE GRAINS, CEREALS*	*PROTEIN*
6 or More Servings*	*5 Servings**	*2–4 Servings**
Strawberries Peppers	Corn	yogurt, sour
Pumpkin	Cornmeal	cream, cot-
Romaine		tage cheese
lettuce		
Spinach		
Squash: acorn,		
butternut		
Sweet potatoes		
Tomatoes		

*A serving is:

1 piece fruit	2 slices bread	3–4 ounces meat, fish, or
½ cup vegetables	2 small muffins	poultry
1 cup fruit juice	1 English muffin	1 egg
	1 bagel	1 cup cooked beans
	½ cup cooked grain	1 8-ounce cup 2% low-fat
	product	milk
		1½ ounces cheese
		1 cup low-fat yogurt
		1 cup cottage cheese

21-DAY MENU PLAN

The following 21-Day Menu Plan incorporates the suggested dietary guidelines made in the report issued by the National Academy of Sciences. Here's how the menus specifically follow the guidelines:

• Americans generally get a large proportion of their daily calories from fat. The report recommended that the proportion be reduced, and that the amount of calories provided by fats should be approximately 30%. Each day's menu derives 30% or fewer of that day's calories from fat.

• The menus include many fruits and vegetables high in Vitamins A and C.

• Cruciferous vegetables are included frequently.

• Whole grain products are included daily.

• There are very few smoked foods on the menus.

• The protein in the menus derives mostly from low-fat food.

Do I have to follow these menus exactly?

You can, if you wish, but my intent is simply that you use these menus as a guide. Look through the menus; eliminate the dishes you really hate, and exchange for your favorites in other daily menus. Substitute from the optional menu in Chapter Fourteen. Or stick as close as possible to guidelines listed for fat, Vitamin A, and Vitamin C. Consult the chart in Chapter Fifteen for detailed nutritional content of the foods you like.

What about calories?

The calorie counts vary. There are a few days when total calories are approximately 1,600, other days when they're around 2,000. Most days fall somewhere between that range. Everyone's need for calories varies. If you're physically active you may need more calories than if you're not. Large-boned, tall people usually need more calories than shorter, fine-boned individuals. You alone can judge how many calories you need to maintain your ideal weight.

How can I increase my caloric intake?

• Add more pasta.

• Add milk to your morning tea or coffee.

• Increase the amount of brown rice, or other whole grain foods.

• Increase the amount of whole wheat breads.
• Add an extra ounce or two to meat, poultry, and fish dishes.
• Add more dried fruits, such as dried apricots.

How can I decrease my caloric intake?

• Eliminate desserts when they're sugar-rich sorbets, sherbets, pies, or cakes.
• Eliminate jams or preserves.
• Cut out canned fruits in thick syrup.
• Substitute fresh fruit or raw vegetables for snacks such as cookies and pound cake.
• Have cantaloupe filled with berries alone, rather than with berries and ice milk.
• Cut down on whole milk products.

Where do I find the recipes for the dishes in the menus?

There is nothing difficult, exotic, or hard-to-find about any of the dishes listed in the 21-Day Menu Plan. All meals are based on recipes easily found in many cookbooks. However, this book includes recipes for those dishes marked with a star.

CHAPTER ELEVEN

WEEK ONE

Monday

NUTRITIONAL INFORMATION:

Total calories: 1,994
Amount of protein (gm.): 90
Amount of fat in (gm.): 54.45
(Less than 30% of total calories)
Vitamin A (IU): 9,860.5
Vitamin C (mg.): 280.6

BREAKFAST:

1 cup orange juice
2 large shredded wheat
  biscuits

1 cup 2% low-fat milk
½ banana
Coffee or tea (optional)

SNACK:

5 prunes

LUNCH:

Turkey (3 ounces
  white meat), lettuce,
  and tomato sandwich
  on whole wheat bread

2 teaspoons mayonnaise
½ cup carrot raisin salad

DINNER:

Cantonese Beef with Radishes and Snow Peas*
½ cup steamed brown rice

1 cup fresh or water-packed pineapple chunks

SNACK:

½ cup 2% low-fat milk

4 ladyfingers topped with ½ cup fresh strawberries

CANTONESE BEEF WITH RADISHES AND SNOW PEAS

3 tablespoons vegetable oil
1 pound flank steak, sliced diagonally into thin strips
6 scallions (green onions), sliced
¼ pound snow peas
12 radishes, sliced

2 tablespoons soy sauce
1 tablespoon brown sugar
2 tablespoons wine vinegar
1 tablespoon cornstarch
½ cup water

Heat 2 tablespoons oil in a large skillet. Add beef and cook for 3 to 5 minutes, or until beef is no longer red. Remove beef from skillet, and reserve.

Heat remaining tablespoon of oil in skillet. Add scallions, snow peas, and radishes. Cook, stirring, for 3 minutes, or until vegetables are hot, and crisply cooked. Remove vegetables from skillet, and reserve.

Off heat add soy sauce, brown sugar, and wine vinegar to skillet, and mix thoroughly. Combine cornstarch and water, mix, and add to skillet. Heat sauce, stirring constantly, until all ingredients are well blended and sauce is hot, thick, and clear.

Return beef and vegetables to skillet, and heat.

Serves: 4

Tuesday

NUTRITIONAL INFORMATION:

Total calories: 1,964
Amount of protein (gm.): 62.5
Amount of fat in (gm.): 49
    (Less than 30% of total calories)
Vitamin A (IU): 10,745
Vitamin C (mg.): 222

BREAKFAST:

1 cup pineapple juice
2 small whole wheat
    pancakes

2 tablespoons maple
    syrup
Coffee or tea (optional)

SNACK:

½ cup raisins

LUNCH:

1 cup Gazpacho*
2 slices pumpernickel
    bread

1½ ounces Swiss cheese
½ cup grapes
1 apple

DINNER:

3 ounces roast leg of
   lamb (lean only)
1 cup brussels sprouts
   (steamed)
½ cup carrots (steamed)

1 baked potato
2 teaspoons sour cream
   and chopped chives
1 small slice lemon
   chiffon pie

SNACK:

1 large pear

GAZPACHO

3 cloves garlic, peeled
1 medium onion,
   peeled and quartered
1 cucumber, peeled
   and quartered
3 ripe tomatoes, peeled
   and quartered
1 green pepper,
   seeded, and cut into
   4 pieces

Dash of cayenne pepper
¼ cup wine vinegar
2 tablespoons olive oil
1 cup tomato juice
¼ teaspoon ground
   cumin
Salt and freshly ground
   black pepper to taste
1 cup croutons

Place garlic, onion, cucumber and tomatoes in a blender, and puree.

Add all remaining ingredients, except for croutons, and blend until everything is liquefied and combined.

Chill soup for one hour before serving, and serve with croutons.

Serves: 4 to 6

Wednesday

NUTRITIONAL INFORMATION:

Total calories: 1,918
Amount of protein (gm.): 97.1
Amount of fat in (gm.): 47:7
(Less than 30% of total calories)
Vitamin A (IU): 5,625
Vitamin C (mg.): 210.5

BREAKFAST:

1 cup cranberry juice
2 small bran muffins
2 pats butter or
   margarine

2 teaspoons jam
Coffee or tea (optional)

SNACK:

½ grapefruit

LUNCH:

Large chef's salad
   containing:
   1 hard-cooked egg, 2
   ounces white meat
   turkey, 1 ounce
   cheddar cheese, 1
   small tomato, ½ small
   cucumber, ½ cup raw
   cauliflower florets, 2
   tablespoons low-calorie
   salad dressing

2 slices whole wheat
   bread
1 fresh or water-packed
   peach

DINNER:

**Spinach noodles with
    skim-milk ricotta and
    tomato sauce**
**Three-bean and tomato
    salad**

**1 slice Italian whole
    wheat bread**
1 cup blueberries

SNACK:

1 cup 2% low-fat milk

**1 whole wheat English
    muffin with 2 teaspoons
    jam**

Thursday

NUTRITIONAL INFORMATION:

Total calories: 1,862
Amount of protein (gm.): 61.8
Amount of fat in (gm.): 59.5
    (Less than 30% of total calories)
Vitamin A (IU): 11,726.5
Vitamin C (mg.): 133.5

BREAKFAST:

1 cup grapefruit juice
**1 cup oatmeal with
    raisins**

Coffee or tea (optional)

SNACK:

1 cup fresh fruit salad   **½ cup low-fat yogurt**

LUNCH:

**Tomato stuffed with egg   2 slices whole wheat
  salad (up to 1   bread
  tablespoon mayonnaise)   1 cup 2% low-fat milk**

DINNER:

**Shrimp Peking*   ½ cup fruit sherbet
½ cup steamed carrots   2 sugar cookies
½ cup steamed brown
  rice**

SNACK:

**2 slices raisin bread   1 teaspoon cinnamon
                                     and sugar**

SHRIMP PEKING

**1 small onion, peeled   1 tablespoon cornstarch
  and thinly sliced   3 tablespoons water
1 clove garlic, pressed   3 tablespoons vegetable
2 tablespoons catsup   oil
2 tablespoons soy sauce   1 pound medium
2 tablespoons wine   shrimp, peeled and
  vinegar   deveined
2 teaspoons brown sugar
1 tablespoon dry Sherry
  wine**

Combine onion, garlic, catsup, soy sauce, wine vinegar, brown sugar, and Sherry wine in a saucepan. Stir, and bring to a simmer over low heat.

Combine cornstarch and water, mixing thoroughly, and add gradually to saucepan, stirring. Cook another minute or two, until sauce thickens and looks clear. Reserve.

Heat oil in a large skillet. Add shrimp, and sauté, stirring, for 4 to 5 minutes, or until shrimp are cooked. Do not overcook, as this toughens the shrimp.

Spoon shrimp onto a serving platter. Reheat sauce for 1 or 2 minutes, and spoon over shrimp.

Serves: 4

Friday

NUTRITIONAL INFORMATION:

Total calories: 1,846
Amount of protein (gm.): 102.9
Amount of fat in (gm.): 367
     (Less than 30% of total calories)
Vitamin A (IU): 16,577.5
Vitamin C (mg.): 178

BREAKFAST:

1 cup grape juice
1 cup whole grain
    ready-to-eat breakfast
    cereal

1 small banana
1 cup 2% low-fat milk
Coffee or tea (optional)

SNACK:

1 cup cherries

LUNCH:

**1 cup low-fat cottage
cheese**
1 cup fresh fruit salad
**2 slices whole wheat
bread**

2 oatmeal cookies
1 cup 2% low-fat milk

DINNER:

**½ dozen clams on the
half shell**
**2 tablespoons cocktail
sauce**
**2 ounces pork roast
(lean only)**

1 baked sweet potato
½ cup broccoli (steamed)
½ cup apple sauce
1 cup gelatin dessert

SNACK:

1 cup popcorn

Saturday

NUTRITIONAL INFORMATION:

Total calories: 2,140.6
Amount of protein (gm.): 83.2
Amount of fat in (gm.): 52.2
    (Less than 30% of total calories)
Vitamin A (IU): 19,136
Vitamin C (mg.): 361.3

BREAKFAST:

1 cup cranberry juice
2 slices Pumpkin
  Bread*
1 pat butter or
  margarine

2 teaspoons jam
½ cup 2% low-fat milk
Coffee or tea (optional)

SNACK:

1 banana

LUNCH:

Antipasto salad:
  1 ounce lean ham
  1 ounce provolone
  1 boiled egg
  1 celery stick
  1 carrot
  2 medium leaves of
    lettuce

  1 tomato
  1 cup mushrooms
  4 black olives
  1 pimiento
2 slices whole wheat
  Italian bread

DINNER:

3 ounces London broil
  (top round)
1 medium baked potato
2 teaspoons sour cream
  and chives
1 stalk broccoli
  (steamed)
1 cup cole slaw with
  mayonnaise-type
  dressing

2 slices whole wheat
  bread
Sponge cake topped
  with crushed pineapple
  (½ cup)

SNACK:

**1 slice watermelon
(or canned water-
packed apricots)**

PUMPKIN BREAD

1 cup sugar	**1 teaspoon baking soda**
2 eggs	**¾ teaspoon salt**
½ cup canned pumpkin	**½ teaspoon cinnamon**
⅓ cup vegetable oil	**¼ teaspoon ground**
1¾ cups all-purpose	**ginger**
flour	

Combine sugar, eggs, pumpkin, and oil in a food processor or an electric mixer, and process or mix thoroughly.

Combine all other ingredients, and add to pumpkin mixture. Mix until ingredients are just combined.

Spoon batter into a nonstick 8-inch loaf pan. Bake in a preheated 350-degree oven for 45 to 50 minutes, or until a toothpick inserted in center of loaf comes out clean.

Yield: 1 loaf
16 slices; 1 slice equals 1 serving

Sunday

NUTRITIONAL INFORMATION:

Total Calories: 2,168
Amount of protein (gm.): 119.2
Amount of fat in (gm.): 74.4
     (Less than 30% of total calories)
Vitamin A (IU): 18,130.5
Vitamin C (mg.): 226.2

BREAKFAST:

½ fresh grapefruit
1 poached egg
2 slices whole wheat
   bread

2 pats butter or
   margarine
2 teaspoons jam
Tea or coffee

SNACK:

1 large orange

LUNCH:

1 whole wheat pita
   bread filled with
   chicken salad (made
   with up to 2 teaspoons
   mayonnaise, herbs
   and spices to taste)

1 ounce Swiss cheese
1 large carrot, 2 stalks
   celery, 4 cherry
   tomatoes
½ cup Fresh Fruit
   Sorbet*

DINNER:

1 serving Flounder Roman Style*	**2 pats butter or margarine**
½ cup steamed cauliflower	**1 small slice angel food cake topped with ½ cup fresh peach slices or berries**
½ cup steamed spinach	
2 slices rye bread	

SNACK:

4 fig bars

FRESH FRUIT SORBET

2½ pounds fresh peaches, plums, or apricots	**1½ cups sugar**
	⅔ cup water
	Juice of 2 lemons

Place your favorite fruit in a large saucepan of boiling water. Cook for 5 minutes, or until fruit can be peeled.

Allow fruit to cool, and peel and pit. Using a blender, food mill, or food processor, puree fruit. You should have 2 cups of fruit puree. Reserve.

Combine sugar and water in a saucepan. Cook, stirring, until mixture comes to a boil. Cook for 2 minutes. Allow syrup to cool for 20 minutes.

Combine fruit puree and sugar syrup, mixing thoroughly. Add lemon juice.

Pour mixture into container of an ice-cream maker, and follow manufacturer's direction.

Serves: 6–8

FLOUNDER ROMAN STYLE

4 **flounder fillets (about 1 pound)**	1 **tablespoon lemon juice**
2 **cloves garlic, pressed**	1 **tablespoon olive oil**
1 **small onion, chopped**	**Salt and freshly ground black pepper to taste**
	½ **cup bread crumbs**

Place fish fillets in a nonstick baking pan. Spoon garlic and onion over fish. Drizzle lemon juice and olive oil over fish, and season. Spoon bread crumbs over all.

Bake fish in a preheated 350-degree oven for 10 minutes, or until fish flakes easily.

Serves: 4

CHAPTER TWELVE

WEEK TWO

Monday

NUTRITIONAL INFORMATION:

Total calories: 1,695
Amount of protein (gm.): 74.6
Amount of fat in (gm.): 54
    (Less than 30% of total calories)
Vitamin A (IU): 9,946
Vitamin C (mg.): 257

BREAKFAST:

1 cup apricot nectar
2 small Cranberry-Apple
    Muffins*
1 pat butter or
    margarine

2 teaspoons jam
Coffee or tea (optional)

SNACK:

1 apple

LUNCH:

Turkey salad (3 ounces
    white meat) with 1
    tablespoon mayonnaise
Lettuce and tomato
2 slices whole wheat
    bread

½ cup cole slaw with
    mayonnaise-type
    dressing
1 banana

DINNER:

1 serving Chicken
 Cacciatora*
½ cup whole wheat
 noodles
½ cup cooked kale

Meringue shells filled
 with ½ cup
 strawberries
1 tablespoon whipped
 cream

SNACK:

1 cup grapes

CRANBERRY-APPLE MUFFINS

1 apple, peeled, cored,
 and finely diced
1 cup fresh
 cranberries, finely
 diced
1 cup sugar

1 egg, lightly beaten
1 cup 2% low-fat milk
2 cups all-purpose flour
1 tablespoon baking
 powder
½ teaspoon salt

Combine apple, cranberries, and sugar in a large bowl;
mix well. Add egg to milk and mix thoroughly. Add
egg-milk mixture to apple-cranberry mixture, and stir.

Combine flour, baking powder, and salt. Add to
apple-milk mixture, and stir to combine thoroughly.

Spoon mixture into 12 greased medium-sized (2¾-inch-
diameter) muffin cups. Cups should be ⅔ full.

Bake in a preheated 400-degree oven for 20 minutes,
or until a toothpick inserted in center of a muffin comes
out clean.

Yield: 12
          1 muffin equals 1 serving

CHICKEN CACCIATORA

1 2½–3-pound chicken,   ½ teaspoon dried basil
  cut into eighths   or 2 tablespoons
2 cups stewed tomatoes   chopped fresh basil
1 clove garlic, minced   Salt and freshly
1 medium onion, sliced   ground black pepper
½ cup dry red wine   to taste

Place chicken pieces in a nonstick baking pan and bake in a preheated 350-degree oven for 20 minutes.

Combine all remaining ingredients in a bowl, and stir to combine.

Pour sauce over chicken, and bake for an additional 20 to 30 minutes, or until chicken is tender.

Serves: 4

Tuesday

NUTRITIONAL INFORMATION:

Total calories: 1,659
Amount of protein (gm.): 57.7
Amount of fat in (gm.): 41
    (Less than 30% of total calories)
Vitamin A (IU): 18,928
Vitamin C (mg.): 298.8

BREAKFAST:

1 cup orange-grapefruit
  juice
2 small bran muffins
1 pat butter or
  margarine

2 teaspoons jam
Coffee or tea (optional)

SNACK:

½ cup 2% low-fat milk

LUNCH:

1 cup tomato juice
2-egg western omelet
2 slices whole wheat
  bread

1 teaspoon jam
Romaine lettuce, orange,
  and red onion salad

DINNER:

Lasagna Vegetarian-
  Style*
Mixed green salad

3 sesame-seed bread
  sticks
1 cup fruit sherbet

SNACK:

1 cup diced mangos (or
  watermelon or canned
  water-packed apricots)

LASAGNA VEGETARIAN-STYLE

1 **package (1 pound) lasagna noodles**
1 **egg, beaten**
1 **pound low-fat ricotta cheese**
2 **teaspoons dried oregano**
1 **clove garlic, pressed**

Salt and freshly ground white pepper to taste
5 **cups tomato sauce**
½ **pound low-fat mozzarella cheese, grated**
½ **cup grated Parmesan cheese**

Cook lasagna noodles *al dente,* or slightly firm to the bite. Drain, and reserve.

Combine egg, ricotta cheese, oregano, garlic, salt and pepper. Mix thoroughly.

Place one layer of lasagna noodles in a baking dish and cover with some of the ricotta mixture, some sauce, mozzarella, and Parmesan cheese.

Repeat layers, until all ingredients are used.

Reserve enough mozzarella cheese and grated Parmesan to top last layer of noodles.

Bake in a preheated 350-degree oven for approximately 20 minutes, or until all ingredients are hot, and mozzarella has melted.

Serves: 8

Wednesday

NUTRITIONAL INFORMATION:

Total calories: 2,067.2
Amount of protein (gm.): 91.7
Amount of fat in (gm.): 40
   (Less than 30% of total calories)
Vitamin A (IU): 31,334.8
Vitamin C (mg.): 284.7

BREAKFAST:

½ cup blueberries
1 cup cream of wheat
½ cup 2% low-fat milk
1 slice whole wheat
   toast

1 pat butter or
   margarine
Coffee or tea (optional)

SNACK:

½ cup dried apricots

LUNCH:

Tex-Mex Chili*
2 small slices corn
   bread

½ cup orange sherbet

DINNER:

3 ounces white meat turkey
1 medium sweet potato
1 slice cranberry sauce
½ cup cauliflower florets (steamed)
2 whole wheat rolls

1 small tomato, sliced
2 teaspoons low-calorie Italian dressing
½ cantaloupe filled with ½ cup ice milk topped with ½ cup berries

SNACK:

2 sugar cookies

½ cup 2% low-fat milk

TEX-MEX CHILI

1 tablespoon olive oil
1 large onion, finely chopped
2 cloves garlic, pressed
1 large green pepper, chopped
3 cups stewed tomatoes
1–2 tablespoons chili powder

½ teaspoon dried cumin
2 tablespoons fresh chopped coriander (cilantro); if coriander isn't available, use parsley
3 cups cooked kidney beans

Heat olive oil in a large skillet or saucepan. Sauté onion, garlic, and green pepper until onion is translucent.

Add tomatoes, chili powder, cumin, and coriander to skillet. Bring sauce to a simmer and stir to combine all ingredients. Cook for 15 minutes over low heat.

Add beans, cover, and cook an additional 30 minutes.
Serves: 4

Thursday

NUTRITIONAL INFORMATION:

Total calories: 1,794
Amount of protein (gm.): 67.1
Amount of fat in (gm.): 61
   (Less than 30% of total calories)
Vitamin A (IU): 12,388
Vitamin C (mg.): 105

BREAKFAST:

1 cup peach nectar
2 small corn muffins
1 pat butter or
   margarine

2 teaspoons strawberry
   preserve
Coffee or tea (optional)

SNACK:

1 cup grapes

LUNCH:

2-egg spinach omelet
2 slices whole wheat
   bread

½ ounce cream cheese
1 cup fruit cocktail
   (water-packed)

DINNER:

1 crock French Onion
   Soup*
Romaine lettuce, orange,
   and red onion salad

2 ounces Swiss or other
   hard cheese
1 apple
½ cup grapes

SNACK:

| 1 slice pound cake | 1 cup 2% low-fat milk |

FRENCH ONION SOUP

4 large onions, peeled and chopped	½ cup dry white wine
1 tablespoon vegetable oil	4 slices French bread, 1 inch thick
1 teaspoon butter	3 ounces grated Swiss cheese
2 teaspoons all-purpose flour	1 tablespoon grated Parmesan cheese
5 cups beef broth	

Heat oil and butter in a large saucepan. Add onions, and cook, stirring from time to time until onions are browned. Be careful not to let onions turn black.

Add flour, and cook, stirring, for an additional 2 to 3 minutes, or until flour has browned slightly.

Gradually add broth and wine, continuing to stir until all ingredients are well blended.

Cover pot, and cook at a low simmer for 30 minutes.

Divide soup into four individual onion soup crocks. Top each crock with 1 bread slice, and sprinkle cheeses on bread slices.

Bake in a preheated 350-degree oven for 10 to 15 minutes, or until cheese has melted and is brown.

Serves: 4

Friday

NUTRITIONAL INFORMATION:

Total calories: 1,828
Amount of protein (gm.): 96.1
Amount of fat in (gm.): 50.2
      (Less than 30% of total calories)
Vitamin A (IU): 16,210.5
Vitamin C (mg.): 204

BREAKFAST:

1 cup grapes
2 slices pumpernickel
  raisin bread

1 ounce cream cheese
Coffee or tea (optional)

SNACK:

½ grapefruit

LUNCH:

2 slices Whole Wheat
  Vegetable Pizza*

Tossed green salad
1 slice honeydew melon

DINNER:

Lemon Baked Chicken*
½ cup each: steamed
  broccoli-cauliflower
  medley

Herbed Brown Rice*
1 slice rye bread
1 slice pumpkin pie

SNACK:

1 ounce hard cheese   1 small apple

WHOLE WHEAT VEGETABLE PIZZA

1 package (¼ ounce)
  active dry yeast
½–1 cup warm water
¼ teaspoon sugar
¾ cup whole wheat
  flour
1 cup all-purpose flour
½ teaspoon salt
¼ teaspoon black
  pepper
1 cup tomato sauce
1 medium zucchini,
  scraped and sliced

1 small onion, peeled
  and chopped
4 ounces low-fat
  mozzarella cheese,
  grated
½ teaspoon dried basil
½ teaspoon dried
  oregano
1 tablespoon grated
  Parmesan cheese

Dissolve yeast in ¼ cup warm water, and stir in sugar. Allow to stand for 5 minutes. Yeast should bubble and grow. If it doesn't, yeast is dead; start again with a fresh package of yeast.

Combine yeast, whole wheat and all-purpose flour, salt and pepper in a large bowl. Work enough of remaining water into dough until dough forms a soft ball.

Remove dough to a lightly floured board, and if necessary add additional flour so that dough is smooth and elastic, and bounces back when it's touched.

Place dough in a floured bowl. Cover, and allow to rise in a warm, draft-free place for 2 to 3 hours, or until dough has doubled in bulk.

Stretch dough to fit a 10-inch pizza pan. Spoon tomato sauce over pizza dough, and top with sliced zucchini and onion. Sprinkle mozzarella cheese and seasonings on top, and add Parmesan cheese.

Bake pizza in a preheated 450-degree oven for 20 minutes, or until crust is brown, vegetables are hot, and cheese has melted.

Serves: 4–8

LEMON BAKED CHICKEN

3 chicken breasts, boned, skin removed, each breast cut in half
2 cloves garlic, pressed
1 small onion, minced
Juice of ½ lemon
½ teaspoon salt (optional)

¼ teaspoon dried basil
¼ teaspoon dried rosemary
¼ teaspoon freshly ground black pepper
1 teaspoon grated Parmesan cheese
½ cup chicken broth

Place chicken pieces in a nonstick baking pan.

Combine all remaining ingredients, stir well, and pour over chicken. Allow chicken to marinate for 1 hour, turning pieces every 20 minutes.

Bake chicken breasts in a preheated 350-degree oven for 20 to 30 minutes, or until chicken is cooked.

Serve with pan juices.

Serves: 6

HERBED BROWN RICE

1 cup uncooked
regular brown rice
2½ cups chicken broth
1 tablespoon chopped
fresh parsley

1 tablespoon chopped
fresh dill
1 tablespoon chopped
fresh chives

Place rice in a large saucepan that has a cover. Bring chicken broth to a boil, and pour over rice.

Cover pot, and cook rice over low heat for 15 minutes. Uncover, and stir in herbs quickly. Cover and continue cooking for 10 to 15 minutes, or until rice is tender and all the liquid has been absorbed.

Serves: 8

Saturday

NUTRITIONAL INFORMATION:

Total calories: 1,782.5
Amount of protein (gm.): 65.3
Amount of fat in (gm): 49.4
(Less than 30% of total calories)
Vitamin A (IU): 18,202
Vitamin C (mg.): 341

BREAKFAST:

2 slices whole wheat
French toast
1 pat butter or
margarine

2 tablespoons maple
syrup
Coffee or tea (optional)

SNACK:

½ grapefruit

LUNCH:

Left-over cold chicken
(3 ounces)
Raw vegetable platter:
  1 small tomato, 1 cup
  cauliflower florets,
  1 cup broccoli florets,
  ¼ cup low-calorie
  dressing

1 whole wheat roll
1 pat butter or
  margarine
1 small slice chocolate
  layer cake

DINNER:

Egg Drop Soup*
Pork Lo Mein*

1 cup canned apricot
  halves in syrup
2 almond cookies

SNACK:

1 orange

EGG DROP SOUP

1 tablespoon vegetable
  oil
¼ pound breast of
  chicken, boned, skin
  removed, chicken cut
  into shreds
4 scallions (green
  onions), chopped
4 cups chicken broth
2 tablespoons corn-
  starch

½ teaspoon sugar
2 teaspoons dry Sherry
  wine
2 teaspoons soy sauce
½ cup finely shredded
  cabbage
2 eggs
¼ cup water

Heat oil in large skillet or saucepan. Add chicken, and sauté, stirring, for 3 minutes, or until chicken is cooked. Add scallions, and sauté, stirring, for another minute. Remove chicken and scallions from skillet and reserve.

Off heat, add the chicken broth, cornstarch, sugar, wine, and soy sauce to skillet. Stir and bring to a simmer. Continue simmering, uncovered, until soup thickens, about 15 minutes. Add shredded cabbage to soup.

Beat eggs with water, and as soup continues to simmer over low heat, pour egg mixture into soup gradually, continuing to stir, so that egg mixture forms thin threads. Return chicken and scallions to soup and simmer an additional 5 minutes.

Serves: 4

PORK LO MEIN

¼ **pound thin spaghetti, or Chinese noodles (vermicelli), cooked**

½ **pound boneless pork loin, cut into thin strips**

3 **tablespoons vegetable oil**

1 **cup chicken broth**

2 **tablespoons soy sauce**

1 **clove garlic, minced**

2 **teaspoons cornstarch**

4 **scallions (green onions), chopped**

2 **tablespoons water**

Salt and freshly ground white pepper to taste

½ **pound Chinese cabbage, cut into thin strips**

Heat 1 tablespoon of oil in a large skillet and sauté garlic and scallions, stirring, for 1 minute. Add Chinese cabbage and cook an additional 2 minutes. Remove vegetables from skillet, and reserve.

Heat remaining oil in skillet and sauté pork, stirring, for 5 to 7 minutes, or until pork is thoroughly cooked.

Return vegetables to skillet. Add chicken broth and soy sauce, and cook, stirring, for 3 minutes.

Combine cornstarch and water in a small bowl, mix well, and add to skillet. Cook, stirring, for another 2 minutes, or until all ingredients are combined.

Add cooked noodles to skillet, toss, and heat until all ingredients are hot.

Serves: 2

Sunday

NUTRITIONAL INFORMATION:

Total calories: 2,251
Amount of protein (gm.): 79.3
Amount of fat in (gm.): 66
    (Less than 30% of total calories)
Vitamin A (IU): 14,264
Vitamin C (mg.): 166.3

BREAKFAST:

½ cantaloupe
1 poached egg
2 slices whole wheat
   toast

1 pat butter or
   margarine
2 teaspoons jam
Coffee or tea (optional)

SNACK:

1 tangerine or orange

LUNCH:

1 serving minestrone soup	3 sesame-seed bread sticks
Cheese board: 1 ounce Swiss, 1 ounce cheddar, 1 ounce provolone	1 pear
	1 apple
	1 cup grapes (or other fruit in season)

DINNER:

Baked Eggplant Parmigiana*	1 pat butter or margarine
1 cup spaghetti with tomato sauce	1 cup fruit sherbet
1 small slice Italian bread	

SNACK:

1 cup 2% low-fat milk

BAKED EGGPLANT PARMIGIANA

1 eggplant (about 1 pound), peeled and cut into ¼-inch slices
½ cup vegetable oil
⅓ cup all-purpose flour
⅓ cup bread crumbs
2 cups tomato sauce
½ teaspoon dried oregano

¼ teaspoon dried basil
Salt and freshly ground black pepper to taste
4 ounces low-fat mozzarella, grated
2 tablespoons grated Parmesan cheese

Dip eggplant slices quickly in and out of oil.

Combine flour and bread crumbs, mix well, and coat eggplant slices with mixture.

Place breaded eggplant slices in a nonstick baking pan, and bake in a preheated 350-degree oven for 15 to 25 minutes, or until eggplant is lightly browned.

Combine tomato sauce with seasonings, and spoon over eggplant. Top with grated cheeses, and return to oven for another 15 minutes, or until cheese has melted and eggplant is tender.

Serves: 6

CHAPTER THIRTEEN

WEEK THREE

Monday

NUTRITIONAL INFORMATION:

Total calories: 1,846
Amount of protein (gm.): 55.68
Amount of fat in (gm.): 33.5
    (Less than 30% of total calories)
Vitamin A (IU): 21,120
Vitamin C (mg.): 181.8

BREAKFAST:

4 stewed prunes
1 whole wheat English
muffin
1 pat butter or
margarine

2 teaspoons jam
Coffee or tea (optional)

SNACK:

1 banana

LUNCH:

Leftover Eggplant
  Parmigiana on whole
  wheat pita bread

Tossed green salad
2 fig bars

DINNER:

3 ounces roast veal
1 serving Stir-Fry
Vegetables*
1 baked potato
1 slice pumpernickel
bread

1 pat butter or
margarine
1 medium orange
2 sugar cookies

SNACK:

1 cup popcorn

STIR-FRY VEGETABLES

2 tablespoons vegetable
oil
1 clove garlic, pressed
2 carrots, sliced
diagonally into ¼ inch
slices
2 celery stalks, sliced
diagonally into ¼ inch
slices
1 onion, thinly sliced
1 8-ounce can water
chestnuts, drained
and sliced

1 medium zucchini,
scraped, sliced
diagonally into ¼ inch
slices
¼ pound mushrooms,
sliced
1 medium tomato, cut
into 6 pieces
2 tablespoons soy
sauce
¼ teaspoon ground
ginger

Heat 1 tablespoon oil in a large skillet. Add garlic, and
stir-fry for 1 minute. Add carrots and celery and stir-fry
for 2 minutes. Add onions and stir-fry for 1 minute.

Add 1 tablespoon oil and water chestnuts, zucchini,

mushrooms, tomato, soy sauce and ginger and stir-fry for 3 minutes. Make sure that all vegetables are thoroughly combined.

Serves: 6

Tuesday

NUTRITIONAL INFORMATION:

Total calories: 1,765.6
Amount of protein (gm.): 73
Amount of fat in (gm.): 57.7
    (Less than 30% of total calories)
Vitamin A (IU): 13,655
Vitamin C (mg.): 255.9

BREAKFAST:

1 cup vanilla yogurt
½ cup sliced fresh
    peaches
2 slices rye bread

1 pat butter or
    margarine
1 teaspoon jam
Coffee or tea (optional)

SNACK:

Carrot and celery sticks

LUNCH:

2 open-face grilled cheese
    and sliced tomato
    sandwiches on whole
    wheat bread (2 slices
    bread total)

½ cup cole slaw with
    mayonnaise
1 slice watermelon (or
    canned, water-packed
    apricots)

DINNER:

Antipasto (1 hard-cooked
    egg, 1 celery stalk,
    1 carrot, sliced, ½
    tomato, sliced, 4 black
    olives, 2 anchovies)
Spaghetti with White
    Clam Sauce*
2 slices whole wheat
    Italian garlic bread,
    made with 1 pat butter
    or margarine

1 large meringue shell
    filled with ½ cup
    berries topped with
    1 tablespoon whipped
    cream

SNACK:

1 cup orange juice

SPAGHETTI WITH WHITE CLAM SAUCE

2 dozen Littleneck
    clams, or 2 cups
    chopped canned clams,
    drained
2 tablespoons olive oil
    or other vegetable oil
4 cloves garlic, pressed
¼ cup chopped fresh
    parsley

¼ cup dry white wine
Salt and freshly ground
    white pepper to taste
1 pound spaghetti (may
    be whole wheat),
    cooked *al dente*

Wash and scrub the clams. Open clams using a clam
knife, or steam open in a small amount of water.

Remove clams from shells, and chop clams coarsely.
Reserve.

Heat oil in a large skillet or saucepan, and add garlic and parsley. Cook, stirring, for 2 to 3 minutes. Add wine, and cook for an additional 2 minutes.

Add clams to skillet, season, and cook for another minute, or until all ingredients are hot. Do not overcook, or clams will toughen.

Pour sauce over cooked spaghetti, and toss to combine.
Serves: 4

Wednesday

NUTRITIONAL INFORMATION:

Total calories: 1,765
Amount of protein (gm.): 67.8
Amount of fat in (gm.): 66.2
      (Less than 30% of total calories)
Vitamin A (IU): 4,824
Vitamin C (mg.): 225

BREAKFAST:

½ cup pineapple chunks
2 small whole wheat
  blueberry muffins

1 pat butter or
  margarine
Coffee or tea (optional)

SNACK:

1 pear

LUNCH:

1 cup turkey noodle
  soup
Cheese, lettuce, and
  tomato sandwich on
  whole wheat bread
  with 1 teaspoon
  mayonnaise

½ cup cole slaw with
  mayonnaise-style
  dressing

DINNER:

2 Chicken Enchiladas
  with Chili Sauce*
Brussels sprouts,
  steamed

Corn on the cob
1 slice sponge cake
  topped with ½ cup ice
  milk

SNACK:

1 cup low-fat yogurt

½ cup raspberries (or
  other berries)

CHICKEN ENCHILADAS WITH CHILI SAUCE

1 small onion, chopped
3 medium tomatoes,
  chopped
1 small green pepper,
  seeded and chopped
1 teaspoon chili
  powder (or more to
  taste)

4 corn tortillas
1 cup cooked diced
  chicken
½ cup shredded
  cabbage
2 tablespoons
  shredded cheddar or
  American cheese

Combine onion, tomatoes, green pepper and chili powder in a saucepan. Cook over low heat, stirring, for five to ten minutes, or until all ingredients are combined and tomatoes have released their juices. Remove from heat and reserve.

Steam tortillas until they are soft. Fill tortillas with chicken and roll. Place seam side down in a shallow baking dish. Pour sauce over all and bake in a 350° pre-heated oven for 15 minutes.

Remove enchiladas and sauce to a serving platter and garnish each enchilada with cabbage and cheese.

Serves: 2–4

Thursday

NUTRITIONAL INFORMATION:

Total calories: 1,583
Amount of protein (gm.): 95.7
Amount of fat in (gm.): 23.9
     (Less than 30% of total calories)
Vitamin A (IU): 13,831
Vitamin C (mg.): 338.5

BREAKFAST:

1 cup cranberry juice
1 serving farina
¼ cup raisins

½ cup 2% low-fat milk
Coffee or tea (optional)

LUNCH:

1 cup low-fat cottage cheese
1 hard cooked egg

Vegetable platter—1 carrot, 4 cherry tomatoes, 2 celery stalks, ½ cup cauliflower florets, ½ cup broccoli florets

SNACK:

½ cup low-fat yogurt

DINNER:

Oriental Pepper Steak*   **2 fortune cookies**
Fried Rice*
**1 cup canned mandarin
   oranges in light syrup**

SNACK:

½ grapefruit

ORIENTAL PEPPER STEAK

2 tablespoons vegetable
  oil
2 cloves garlic, finely
  minced
1 slice fresh ginger
  root, cut ¼ inch thick,
  finely minced
1 large onion, thinly
  sliced
2 large green peppers,
  cored, seeded, and
  sliced into thin strips
1½ pound flank steak,
  sliced diagonally into
  thin strips

2 medium tomatoes,
  quartered
1½ cups beef broth
2 tablespoons dry
  Sherry wine
2 tablespoons soy
  sauce
½ teaspoon dark
  brown sugar
1 tablespoon corn
  starch

Heat 1 tablespoon oil in a large skillet. Add garlic and ginger root to skillet, and cook stirring, for 1 minute.

Add onion and green pepper, and cook, stirring, for an additional 2 minutes. Remove all ingredients from skillet and reserve.

Heat remaining oil in skillet and add steak slices. Cook, stirring, for 2 minutes. Add tomato, and cook an additional minute. Remove ingredients from skillet, and reserve.

Combine all remaining ingredients in a bowl, and blend thoroughly. Pour into skillet, and cook, stirring constantly, until sauce is hot, thick, and clear.

Return all ingredients to sauce in skillet, and cook, stirring until everything is thoroughly combined and hot.

Serves: 6

FRIED RICE

2 tablespoons vegetable oil

6 scallions (green onions) chopped

6 medium shrimp, cleaned, cooked, and chopped

1 cup cooked peas

3 cups cooked brown rice

½ cup soy sauce

2 eggs, well beaten

Heat 1 tablespoon oil in a large skillet, or nonstick pan. Add scallions, and cook, stirring, for 2 minutes. Add shrimp and peas, and cook, stirring for an additional 2 minutes. Remove all ingredients from skillet.

Heat remaining tablespoon oil in skillet and add rice. Heat, stirring, until rice is thoroughly hot. Return vegetables and shrimp to skillet, and fold into rice. Add soy sauce to skillet, stirring.

Quickly blend in beaten eggs, and cook, stirring, until eggs set, about 2 minutes, and all ingredients are hot.

Serves: 6

Friday

NUTRITIONAL INFORMATION:

Total calories: 1,785
Amount of protein (gm.): 101.3
Amount of fat in (gm.): 64.7
    (Less than 30% of total calories)
Vitamin A (IU): 17,335
Vitamin C (mg.): 125.5

BREAKFAST:

1 slice honeydew melon
3 small buckwheat
    pancakes

1 tablespoon jam
Coffee or tea (optional)

SNACK:

1 hard-cooked egg

LUNCH:

Tomato stuffed with
    chicken salad made
    with 3 ounces white
    chicken and 1
    tablespoon mayonnaise

2 slices whole wheat
    bread
1 pat butter or
    margarine

DINNER:

1 cup Manhattan clam chowder	½ cup kale
	½ cup carrot puree
Baked flounder or cod	1 slice lemon chiffon pie

SNACK:

1 cup 2% low-fat milk

Saturday

NUTRITIONAL INFORMATION:

Total calories: 1,621.5
Amount of protein (gm.): 85.3
Amount of fat in (gm.): 55.2
    (Less than 30% of total calories)
Vitamin A (IU): 8,511
Vitamin C (mg.): 169

BREAKFAST:

1 cup low-fat cottage cheese	1 slice whole wheat bread
½ cup fresh peach slices	1 pat butter or margarine
1 slice pineapple	Coffee or tea (optional)

SNACK:

1 hard-cooked egg

LUNCH:

2 ounces lean ham, 1
ounce Swiss cheese,
and lettuce and tomato
on 2 slices whole wheat
bread

1 apple

DINNER:

Fettucini with Pesto
Sauce*
1 yellow cupcake with
chocolate icing

1 cup 2% low-fat milk

SNACK:

1 slice watermelon (or
1 cup canned, water-
packed apricots)

FETTUCINE WITH PESTO SAUCE

2 cups, packed, fresh
basil leaves
2 cloves garlic
½ cup low-fat ricotta
cheese

¼ cup grated
Parmesan cheese
2 tablespoons olive oil
1 pound fettucine
noodles

Place all ingredients, except for noodles, in a food
processor or blender. Process until all ingredients are a
smooth puree. Reserve.

Cook fettucine noodles until they are *al dente,* or
slightly firm to the bite.

Remove ¼ cup of cooking water from noodles and add to pesto sauce; stir to combine.

Drain fettucine noodles, and pour sauce over noodles. Toss, and serve immediately. This dish can also be prepared in advance, and served 2 to 3 hours later. Serve at room temperature; do not reheat.

Serves: 4

Sunday

NUTRITIONAL INFORMATION:

Total calories: 1,752.5
Amount of protein (gm.): 67.6
Amount of fat in (gm.): 55.8
   (Less than 30% of total calories)
Vitamin A (IU): 18,790
Vitamin C (mg.): 221

BREAKFAST:

1 cup fresh fruit cocktail
2 slices raisin toast
1 pat butter or
   margarine

1 teaspoon cinnamon
   sugar
Coffee or tea (optional)

SNACK:

1 carrot

1 celery stalk

LUNCH:

1 cup split pea soup
Green salad with
   oranges and red onions

2 whole wheat rolls
1 piece watermelon

DINNER:

3 ounces roast beef au
   jus (lean only)
1 medium baked potato
2 teaspoons sour cream

½ cup brussels sprouts
1 serving Spinach Salad*
1 slice Pound Cake
1 cup 2% low-fat milk

SNACK:

1 apple

SPINACH SALAD

3 slices bacon, cooked
   until crisp, and
   crumbled
3 cups raw spinach,
   washed
1 cup sliced raw
   mushrooms

1 large tomato cut
   into 6 pieces
2 tablespoons low-
   calorie Italian salad
   dressing

Divide spinach, mushrooms, and tomatoes into three
equal servings. Sprinkle with bacon. Spoon salad dressing equally over each portion.
   Serves: 3

CHAPTER FOURTEEN

A WEEK OF OPTIONAL MENUS

Monday

BREAKFAST:

1 cup pineapple-
  grapefruit juice
1 whole wheat bagel

1 ounce cream cheese
Coffee or tea (optional)

SNACK:

1 medium banana

LUNCH:

4 ounces lean
  hamburger on whole
  wheat English muffin
Lettuce, tomato, red
  onion salad

Corn on the cob
Cole slaw

DINNER:

1 serving lentil soup
  with barley
1 serving poached
  salmon with spinach
  or kale sauce

½ cup Bulgur Salad
  (Tabbouleh)*
½ cup broccoli
1 slice angel food cake

SNACK:

½ cup applesauce

BULGUR SALAD (Tabbouleh)

2 cups (½ pound)
uncooked bulgur

2 scallions (green
onions) minced

4 tablespoons parsley,
minced

2 tablespoons dried
crushed mint, or 3
tablespoons minced
fresh mint

5 tablespoons olive oil

5 tablespoons lemon
juice

Salt and freshly ground
black pepper to taste

Cabbage leaves, tender,
uncooked

Place bulgur in a large bowl, and pour boiling water
over it to cover. Let stand for 1 hour. Bulgur will swell
as it absorbs water. Drain bulgur, and squeeze out as
much water as possible with your hands.

Spread bulgur on a cloth, and allow to dry for an
additional 15 minutes.

Return bulgur to bowl, and add all other ingredients
except cabbage. Mix thoroughly and chill for at least 1
hour before serving.

Serve bulgur salad with cabbage leaves, which are
used to scoop up the bulgur and are eaten along with the
salad.

Serves: 8

Tuesday

BREAKFAST:

1 cup cranapple juice
2 slices date-nut bread
1 tablespoon cream
   cheese

Coffee or tea (optional)

SNACK:

1 slice whole wheat
   bread with 2 teaspoons
   peanut butter

LUNCH:

Pita Bread Vegetable
   Hero Sandwich*

Tossed green salad with
   1 tablespoon low
   calorie dressing

DINNER:

Stuffed breast of veal
Puree of Kale and
   Potatoes*
½ cup carrots, steamed

2 small corn muffins
2 pats butter or
   margarine

SNACK:

Frozen yogurt on a cone

PITA BREAD VEGETABLE HERO SANDWICHES

1 tomato, sliced
1 tablespoon olive oil
   or other vegetable oil
¼ cup bean sprouts
1 cup shredded cabbage
4 scallions (green
   onions), chopped
1 small red onion,
   sliced

1 small cucumber,
   sliced
¼ cup shredded
   cheese (cheddar,
   American, or goat
   cheese)
2 whole wheat pita
   breads

Carefully separate each pita bread partially, creating a pocket in each bread.

Sprinkle tomato slices with oil, and place half of tomato slices in each pita bread. Top with all other ingredients.

Serves: 2

PUREE OF KALE AND POTATOES

1 bunch kale (about ½
   pound)
2 large potatoes,
   peeled, cooked, and
   mashed
2 tablespoons butter or
   margarine

¼ cup low-fat plain
   yogurt
1 egg, lightly beaten
Salt and freshly
   ground black pepper
   to taste

Wash kale, and snap off stems and discard.

Steam, or cook kale in water to cover, for approximately 5 to 10 minutes, or until vegetable is tender. Drain.

Using a food processor or food mill, puree kale.

Combine kale, potatoes, and butter, mixing thoroughly. Stir in yogurt, mix again, and add egg and seasonings, stirring until all ingredients are thoroughly combined.

Spoon kale-potato puree into an ovenproof baking dish, and bake in a preheated 350-degree oven for 15 to 20 minutes, or until puree is hot and top is lightly browned.

Serves: 3–4

Wednesday

BREAKFAST:

1 cup orange juice   ½ cup 2% low-fat milk
1 cup oatmeal   Coffee or tea (optional)

SNACK:

6 dried apricots

LUNCH:

1 cup cream of carrot   1 slice sponge cake
  soup   topped with ½ cup
Broiled filet of sole   sliced strawberries
Tossed green salad

DINNER:

Bulgar Pilaf and Lamb*   2 pats butter or
1 cup string beans   margarine
2 small slices whole
  wheat Italian bread

SNACK:

1 apple

BULGUR PILAF AND LAMB

1 cup bulgur
1 tablespoon vegetable oil
1 small onion, minced
1 pound lean ground lamb
¼ cup pignolia (pine nuts)

Salt and freshly ground black pepper to taste
¼ teaspoon ground cumin

Place bulgur in a bowl and pour on enough boiling water to cover. Let stand for 30 minutes.

Heat oil in a skillet and sauté onion for 3 minutes, stirring. Add ½ pound of lamb to skillet, and cook, stirring, for 10 minutes. Add pignolia nuts and salt and pepper; stir to combine. Reserve.

Drain bulgur, and squeeze excess water out of bulgur with your hands. Add remaining ½ pound of lamb and cumin to bulgur, and mix thoroughly.

Spread half of bulgur-lamb mixture on bottom of a baking dish. Top with all of the lamb-nut mixture, and cover with the other half of the bulgur-lamb mixture.

Place in a preheated 350-degree oven and bake for 50 to 60 minutes, or until top is brown and crusty. To serve, cut into squares.

Serves: 8

Thursday

BREAKFAST:

1 cup orange-pineapple
  juice
1 whole wheat roll

2 teaspoons cream
  cheese
Coffee or tea (optional)

SNACK:

½ cup raisins

LUNCH:

1 cup tomato juice
Vegetable quiche

DINNER:

Baked stuffed pork
  chops
Corn on the cob
1 slice whole wheat
  bread

Home-Style Cole Slaw*
Peach tart
1 cup 2% low-fat milk

SNACK:

1 cup granola

HOME-STYLE COLE SLAW

1 head of cabbage
   (about 1½–2 pounds),
   shredded
1 carrot, sliced
1 green pepper, cored,
   seeded, and coarsely
   chopped
1 small onion, grated
1 cup low-calorie
   mayonnaise

2 tablespoons white
   vinegar
¼ cup 2% low-fat
   milk
Salt and freshly
   ground black pepper
   to taste
2 teaspoons sugar (or to
   taste)

Combine cabbage, carrot, green pepper, and onion, mixing thoroughly. Reserve.

Combine all other ingredients, blending thoroughly. Spoon over cabbage mixture, and toss to combine.

Serves: 6–8

Friday

BREAKFAST:

1 cup orange juice
2 scones
1 pat butter or
   margarine

2 teaspoons jam

SNACK:

1 plum

LUNCH:

2 deviled eggs
Raw vegetable platter:
  1 carrot, 1 cup
  cauliflower flowerets,
  1 cup broccoli
  flowerets, 2 stalks
  celery

¼ cup low-calorie dip
  (such as Avocado Dip*
  or East Indian Dip*)
4 sesame-seed bread
  sticks

DINNER:

Stuffed Cabbage in
  Tomato Sauce with
  Brown Rice*

2 small slices Italian
  whole wheat bread
Cantaloupe

SNACK:

½ cup ice milk

AVOCADO DIP

1 avocado, peeled and
  seeded
1 cup low-fat yogurt
2 teaspoons lemon juice
½ teaspoon salt
  (optional)

⅛ teaspoon ground
  cumin
¼ teaspoon hot
  pepper sauce

Combine all ingredients in a blender or food processor, and puree until smooth. Chill for at least half an hour, and serve with raw vegetables.

    Yield: 1½–2 cups, approximately

EAST INDIAN DIP

1 small cucumber,
  peeled and shredded
1 small onion, peeled
  and shredded
2 cups low-fat plain
  yogurt

1 garlic clove, pressed
1 teaspoon ground
  cumin
Salt and freshly
  ground white pepper
  to taste

Combine all ingredients in a bowl, mixing thoroughly.
  Chill for 1 hour, and serve with raw vegetables.
  Yield: 2 cups, approximately

STUFFED CABBAGE IN TOMATO SAUCE
WITH BROWN RICE

1 head of cabbage
  (about 2 pounds)
1 pound ground veal
1 cup cooked brown
  rice
2 cloves garlic,
  pressed

1 egg, lightly beaten
1/8 teaspoon ground
  cumin (optional)
Salt and freshly ground
  black pepper to taste
1 cup tomato sauce
2 cups beef broth

Parboil cabbage in boiling water for 5 minutes. Drain
and allow to cool.
  Turn the cabbage upside down and cut out the core.
Turn cabbage right side up, and carefully pull the cabbage leaves apart, working from the center, until there
is a hollow formed within the cabbage. Reserve cabbage.
  Combine veal, rice, garlic, egg, and seasonings. Mix
thoroughly.
  Remove 2 large outside leaves from cabbage and

reserve. Stuff meat mixture into the center of the cabbage, and place the reserved leaves on top. Tie cabbage around with butcher's string, and place stuffed cabbage in an ovenproof baking dish or casserole that has a cover.

Combine tomato sauce and beef broth in a saucepan, and bring to a simmer, stirring. Pour tomato-beef broth sauce over and around the cabbage.

Cover dish, and bake cabbage in a 350-degree preheated oven for 1½ to 2 hours, or until cabbage is tender and meat is cooked.

Serves: 6

Saturday

BREAKFAST:

1 cup vanilla low-fat yogurt

1 cup fresh fruit cocktail

1 whole wheat English muffin

2 teaspoons jam

Coffee or tea (optional)

SNACK:

1 cup popcorn

LUNCH:

Spring salad sandwich on whole wheat bread (chopped scallions, carrots, cucumber, and tomato)

DINNER:

Chickpea and Sesame
 Appetizer*
Broccoli and Pasta*
Roast chicken
2 small slices whole
 wheat Italian bread

1 pat butter or
 margarine
Fresh fruit sorbet

CHICKPEA AND SESAME APPETIZER

2 cups cooked chickpeas
1 tablespoon olive oil
Juice of 1 lemon
1 clove garlic, pressed
½ cup sesame-seed paste
 (also known as tahini)

½–¾ cup water
Salt and freshly ground
 white pepper to taste

Using a food mill or a food processor, puree chickpeas. Add olive oil, lemon juice, and garlic and mix. Gradually stir in sesame-seed paste, making sure all ingredients are well combined.

Add water gradually. Mixture should be a thick, creamy mass, and liquid enough to be used as a dip. Season to taste.

Spoon puree into a bowl, and serve with small wedges of whole wheat pita bread, carrot sticks, and cherry tomatoes which have been cut in half.

Serves: 6

BROCCOLI AND PASTA

1 bunch broccoli (about
   1½ pounds)
2 tablespoons olive oil
2 tomatoes, peeled
   and finely chopped
1 clove garlic, pressed
   (optional)

1 pound pasta:
   linguine or thin
   spaghetti (may be
   whole wheat pasta)
Salt and freshly
   ground black pepper
   to taste

Wash broccoli. Cut off lower parts of the stalks and discard.

Steam, or cook broccoli in boiling water to cover, until vegetable is tender but not limp, about 15 minutes. Drain and allow to cool.

In a large, nonstick pan, heat olive oil, and add tomatoes and garlic to pan. Cook, stirring, for 5 minutes, over low heat.

Cut broccoli stalks into 2–3-inch pieces and add to pan. Cook, stirring, for 2 to 3 minutes, and remove from heat. Reserve.

Cook pasta until *al dente,* or slightly firm to the bite. Drain. Spoon broccoli sauce over pasta and toss to combine all ingredients.

Serves: 4–6

Sunday

BREAKFAST:

1 cup apple cider
1 buckwheat waffle
1 teaspoon honey
½ cup sliced
   strawberries

1 tablespoon sour
   cream
Coffee or tea, optional

LUNCH:

Cold left-over roast chicken
Sliced tomatoes

Small whole wheat roll
1 pat butter or margarine

SNACK:

6 dried apricots

DINNER:

1 Vegetable Shish Kebab*
1 cup herbed brown rice

1 medium banana, sliced, topped with 1 teaspoon chocolate syrup and 2 teaspoons whipped cream

SNACK:

1 orange

VEGETABLE SHISH KEBAB

2 cups vegetable broth or bouillon
½ cup soy sauce
2 tablespoons vegetable oil
1 clove garlic, pressed
¼ teaspoon ground cinnamon
Freshly ground black pepper to taste
8 2-inch cubes firm tofu (bean curd)

2 green peppers, seeded and cut into quarters
2 small sweet potatoes, peeled and cut into ½-inch slices
2 tomatoes, quartered
1 large onion, quartered
4 large mushroom caps
2 small zucchini, scraped and cut into 3-inch pieces

Prepare marinade by combining vegetable broth, soy sauce, vegetable oil, garlic, cinnamon, and black pepper in a small saucepan. Bring ingredients to a simmer, stirring, and cook for 3 minutes.

Drain tofu cubes and place in a shallow dish. Pour hot marinade over tofu and cover. Refrigerate for 8 hours.

Remove tofu from marinade, and reserve marinade. Using 1 skewer for each serving, alternate tofu and vegetables on skewers.

Brush marinade over skewered ingredients and broil or barbecue for approximately 10 minutes, or until vegetables and tofu are browned and hot. Serve with brown rice.

Serves: 4

CHAPTER FIFTEEN

ADDITIONAL FACTS AND MANY MORE OPTIONS

You've now read the 21-day Menu Plan, and that, plus the dietary guidelines you've read before, may have you wondering about the following:

What about additives? Is it important to avoid them?

It's hard to avoid additives, because according to the report, almost 3000 substances are added to processed foods. And these are just the direct additives. Then there are the 12,000 chemicals used in packaging foods, which are considered indirect additives.

Sugar, which the committee considers an additive (it's found in baked goods, ice cream, bottled sauces, dressings, canned fruits) is eaten in large quantities by most of us, but other additives play only a tiny part in our diet.

Some direct food additives have been tested, and when they've been found to be carcinogenic to animals they've been banned from use. The one exception to this is saccharin, which has not been banned.

However, there haven't been very many studies done using groups of people to examine the possibility of a relationship between additives and cancer, and right now there is no scientific evidence indicating that the use of food additives has increased the risk of cancer. This may be because the additives aren't carcinogenic, or because they haven't been studied sufficiently. Says the committee, ". . . no definitive conclusion can be reached until more data become available."

If fats are so bad, why not cut them down to 10% of the day's diet, or eliminate them completely?

The Lifelong Anti-Cancer Diet has stressed moderation on almost every page. Fats should not be eliminated entirely, or even cut down too drastically, because Vitamins A, D, E, and K are fat-soluble vitamins, and your body won't be able to absorb them without a certain amount of fat. In addition, a recent medical report on running has indicated that many athletes who cut down too far on fats became seriously ill during or after racing. Too much fat is bad for the heart, but without fat, the heart cannot function.

The menus call for butter or margarine. Isn't polyunsaturated margarine better?

The report recommends reducing the amount of all fats in the diet, not saturated fats in particular. And in laboratory studies with animals there has been some evidence that in a low-fat diet, polyunsaturated fats are more effective than saturated fats in promoting tumor formation. If there are other health reasons for you to stick to polyunsaturates, do so.

The 21-Day Menu Plan seems very low in protein, at least compared to other diets I've been on. Why is that?

There have been many popular diets stressing high protein. However, the Recommended Daily Dietary Allowance (RDA) for protein, as advised by the National Research Council of the National Academy of Sciences, ranges between 44 and 56 grams, depending on age and sex, and the 21-Day Menu Plan has that, and usually more, every day.

Protein is a most necessary nutrient: It helps produce antibodies needed to fight infection, has been called one of the building blocks of the body, aids in the mechanical action of muscles, and contributes to the elasticity of blood vessels.

However, once that has been said, it's important to know that most Americans eat two to five times their minimum protein requirement, and much of that protein is associated with fat. Possibly you've been on a high-protein diet, but the 21-Day Menu Plan is not low in protein when compared to the RDA.

If I create my own plan, how can I figure out the percentage of fats in my diet?

To figure out the percentage of fat in your daily diet, do the following:

• Add the grams of fat you've eaten in one day. Multiply that number by 9, because there are 9 calories in each gram of fat. You now have the number of calories derived from fat.

• Total the calories you've eaten the same day.

• Now, figure out the percentage of fat calories to total calories. (*Example*: Let's say you've had 40 grams of fat in one day. Multiplied by 9, that equals 360 calories derived from fat. Now let's say your total caloric intake for the same day was 1,800. 30% of that would be 540 calories, so your fat intake of 360 calories was well within recommended limits.)

I'd like to figure out the percentage of protein in my daily diet. How do I do that?

Follow the directions for figuring the percentage of fat in the diet, except multiply each gram of protein by 4.

Do I have to eat cruciferous vegetables every day?

If you want to, by all means eat cruciferous vegetables every day, but if you don't, understand that this is a *lifelong plan*. If you skip a day or even several days, don't abandon the plan; just try to include more of the items you've been neglecting in future meals. This applies to all foods, not only cruciferous vegetables.

How can I create a menu plan that would be more pleasing to me?

If you want an alternative to the 21-Day Menu Plan you can create your own individual plan by following the dietary guidelines and recommendations listed in Chapter 10 and elsewhere in the book, and by paying special attention to the Chart of Foods to be included in the Daily Diet, also in Chapter 10.

How can I extend the diet plan past 21 days?

To successfully create original meals and menus that follow the dietary guidelines it's important to know certain nutritive values of foods. The following charts are based on information from the United States Department of Agriculture. Consult them when you want to eat foods that are not included in the 21-Day Plan.

Nutritive values do vary, however, especially in packaged foods. Some products are enriched with vitamins, while others are not. Read the labels of packaged goods for accuracy. Nutritive values in produce may also vary, depending on the variety of the produce and the season in which they're grown.

NUTRITIVE VALUES IN FREQUENTLY EATEN FOODS

DAIRY PRODUCTS (CHEESE, CREAM, IMITATION CREAM, MILK; RELATED PRODUCTS)

Butter. See Fats, oils; related products.

		Grams	Cal.	Pro. (gm.)	Fat (gm.)	A (IU)	C (IU)
Cheese:							
Natural:							
Blue	1 oz	28	100	6	8	200	0
Camembert (3 wedges per 4-oz container).	1 wedge	38	115	8	9	350	0
Cheddar:							
Cut pieces	1 oz	28	115	7	9	300	0
	1 cu in	17.2	70	4	6	180	0
Shredded	1 cup	113	455	28	37	1,200	0
Cottage (curd not pressed down):							
Creamed (cottage cheese, 4% fat):							
Large curd	1 cup	225	235	28	10	370	Trace
Small curd	1 cup	210	220	26	9	340	Trace

DAIRY PRODUCTS (CHEESE, CREAM, IMITATION CREAM, MILK; RELATED PRODUCTS) Cont.

		Grams	Cal.	Pro. (gm.)	Fat (gm.)	A (IU)	C (IU)
Low fat (2%)	1 cup	226	205	31	4	160	Trace
Low fat (1%)	1 cup	226	165	28	2	80	Trace
Uncreamed (cottage cheese dry curd, less than ½% fat).	1 cup	145	125	25	1	40	0
Cream	1 oz	28	100	2	10	400	0
Mozzarella, made with—							
Whole milk	1 oz	28	90	6	7	260	0
Part skim milk	1 oz	28	80	8	5	180	0
Parmesan, grated:							
Cup, not pressed down	1 cup	100	455	42	30	700	0
Tablespoon	1 tbsp	5	25	2	2	40	0
Ounce	1 oz	28	130	12	9	200	0
Provolone	1 oz	28	100	7	8	230	0
Ricotta, made with—							
Whole milk	1 cup	246	430	28	32	1,210	0
Part skim milk	1 cup	246	340	28	19	1,060	0
Romano	1 oz	28	110	9	8	160	0
Swiss	1 oz	28	105	8	8	240	0
Pasteurized process cheese:							
American	1 oz	28	105	6	9	340	0

Food	Measure	Grams	Calories				
Swiss	1 oz	28	95	7	7	230	0
Pasteurized process cheese food, American.	1 oz	28	95	6	7	260	0
Pasteurized process cheese spread, American.	1 oz	28	80	5	6	220	0
Cream, sweet:							
Half-and-half (cream and milk)	1 cup	242	315	7	28	260	2
	1 tbsp	15	20	Trace	2	20	Trace
Light, coffee, or table	1 cup	240	470	6	46	1,730	2
	1 tbsp	15	30	Trace	3	110	Trace
Whipping, unwhipped (volume about double when whipped):							
Light	1 cup	239	700	5	74	2,690	1
	1 tbsp	15	45	Trace	5	170	Trace
Heavy	1 cup	238	820	5	88	3,500	1
	1 tbsp	15	80	Trace	6	220	Trace
Whipped topping, (pressurized)-	1 cup	60	155	2	13	550	0
	1 tbsp	3	10	Trace	1	30	0
Cream, sour	1 cup	230	495	7	48	1,820	2
	1 tbsp	12	25	Trace	3	90	Trace

DAIRY PRODUCTS (CHEESE, CREAM, IMITATION CREAM, MILK; RELATED PRODUCTS) Cont.

		Grams	Cal.	Pro. (gm.)	Fat (gm.)	A (IU)	C (IU)
Cream products, imitation (made with vegetable fat):							
Sweet:							
Creamers:							
Liquid (frozen)	1 cup	245	335	2	24	[1]220	0
	1 tbsp	15	20	Trace	1	[1]10	0
Powdered	1 cup	94	515	5	33	[1]190	0
	1 tsp	2	10	Trace	1	[1]Trace	0
Whipped topping:							
Frozen	1 cup	75	240	1	19	[1]650	0
	1 tbsp	4	15	Trace	1	[1]30	0
Powdered, made with whole milk.	1 cup	80	150	3	10	[1]290	1
	1 tbsp	4	10	Trace	Trace	[1]10	Trace
Pressurized	1 cup	70	185	1	16	[1]330	0
	1 tbsp	4	10	Trace	1	[1]20	0
Sour dressing (imitation sour cream) made with nonfat dry milk.	1 cup	235	415	8	39	[1]20	2
	1 tbsp	12	20	Trace	2	[1]Trace	Trace

Ice cream. See Milk desserts, frozen

Ice milk. See Milk desserts, frozen

Milk:

Fluid:

Whole (3.3% fat)	1 cup	244	150	8	8	²310	2
Lowfat (2%):							
No milk solids added	1 cup	244	120	8	5	500	2
Milk solids added:							
Label claim less than 10 g of protein per cup.	1 cup	245	125	9	5	500	2
Label claim 10 or more grams of protein per cup (protein fortified).	1 cup	246	135	10	5	500	3
Lowfat (1%):							
No milk solids added	1 cup	244	100	8	3	500	2
Milk solids added:							
Label claim less than 10 g of protein per cup.	1 cup	245	105	9	2	500	2

[1] Applies to product without Vitamin A added.
[2] Applies to product with added Vitamin A. Without added Vitamin A, value is 20 International Units (IU).

DAIRY PRODUCTS (CHEESE, CREAM, IMITATION CREAM, MILK; RELATED PRODUCTS) Cont.

	Grams	Cal.	Pro. (gm.)	Fat (gm.)	A (IU)	C (IU)
Label claim 10 or more grams of protein per cup (protein fortified). 1 cup	246	120	10	3	500	3
Nonfat (skim):						
No milk solids added 1 cup	245	85	8	Trace	500	2
Milk solids added:						
Label claim less than 10 g of protein per cup. 1 cup	245	90	9	1	500	2
Label claim 10 or more grams of protein per cup (protein fortified). 1 cup	246	100	10	1	500	3
Buttermilk 1 cup	245	100	8	2	[1]80	2
Canned:						
Evaporated, unsweetened:						
Whole milk 1 cup	252	340	17	19	[1]610	5
Skim milk 1 cup	255	200	19	1	[2]1,000	3
Sweetened, condensed 1 cup	306	980	24	27	[1]1,000	8
Dried:						
Buttermilk 1 cup	120	465	41	7	[1]260	7

Nonfat instant:							
Envelope, net wt., 3.2 oz[3]-1 envelope		91	325	32	1	[4]2,160	5
Cup[5]	1 cup	68	245	24	Trace	[4]1,610	4
Milk beverages:							
Chocolate milk (commercial):							
Regular	1 cup	250	210	8	8	[1]300	2
Lowfat (2%)	1 cup	250	180	8	5	500	2
Lowfat (1%)	1 cup	250	160	8	3	500	2
Eggnog (commercial)	1 cup	254	340	10	19	890	4
Malted milk, home-prepared with 1 cup of whole milk and 2 to 3 heaping tsp of malted milk powder (about ¾ oz):							
Chocolate	1 cup of milk plus ¾ oz of powder.	265	235	9	9	330	2
Natural	1 cup of milk plus ¾ oz of powder.	265	235	11	10	380	2

[1]Applies to product without Vitamin A added.
[2]Applies to product with added Vitamin A. Without added Vitamin A, value is 20 International Units (IU).
[3]Yields 1 qt. of fluid milk when reconstituted according to package directions.
[4]Applies to product with added Vitamin A.
[5]Weight applies to product with label claim of 1⅓ cups equal 3.2 oz.

DAIRY PRODUCTS (CHEESE, CREAM, IMITATION CREAM, MILK; RELATED PRODUCTS) Cont.

		Grams	Cal.	Pro. (gm.)	Fat (gm.)	A (IU)	C (IU)
Shakes, thick:[6]							
Chocolate, container, net wt., 10.6 oz.	1 container	300	355	9	8	260	0
Vanilla, container, net wt., 11 oz.	1 container	313	350	12	9	360	0
Milk desserts, frozen:							
Ice cream:							
Regular (about 11% fat):							
Hardened	½ gal	1,064	2,155	38	115	4,340	6
	1 cup	133	270	5	14	540	1
	3-fl oz container	50	100	2	5	200	trace
Soft serve (frozen custard)	1 cup	173	375	7	23	790	1
Rich (about 16% fat), hardened.	½ gal	1,188	2,805	33	190	7,200	5
	1 cup	148	350	4	24	900	1
Ice milk:							
Hardened (about 4.3% fat)	½ gal	1,048	1,470	41	45	1,710	6
	1 cup	131	185	5	6	210	1
Soft serve (about 2.6 % fat)	1 cup	175	225	8	5	180	1
Sherbet (about 2% fat)	½ gal	1,542	2,160	17	31	1,480	31
	1 cup	193	270	2	4	190	4

Milk desserts, other:							
Custard, baked	1 cup	265	305	14	15	930	1
Puddings:							
From home recipe:							
Starch base:							
Chocolate	1 cup	260	385	8	12	390	1
Vanilla (blancmange)	1 cup	255	285	9	10	410	2
Tapioca cream	1 cup	165	220	8	8	480	2
From mix (chocolate) and milk:							
Regular (cooked)	1 cup	260	320	9	8	340	2
Instant	1 cup	260	325	8	7	340	2
Yogurt:							
With added milk solids:							
Made with low-fat milk:							
Fruit-flavored	1 container, net wt., 8 oz	227	230	10	3	120	1
Plain	1 container, net wt., 8 oz	227	145	12	4	150	2
Made with nonfat milk	1 container, net wt., 8 oz	227	125	13	trace	20	2
Without added milk solids:							
Made with whole milk	1 container, net wt., 8 oz	227	140	8	7	280	1

⁶Applies to products made from thick shake mixes and that do not contain added ice cream. Products made from milk shake mixes are higher in fat and usually contain added ice cream.

EGGS

		Grams	Cal.	Pro. (gm.)	Fat (gm.)	A (IU)	C (IU)
Eggs, large (24 oz per dozen):							
Raw:							
Whole, without shell	1 egg	50	80	6	6	260	0
White	1 white	33	15	3	trace	0	0
Yolk	1 yolk	17	65	3	6	310	0
Cooked:							
Fried in butter	1 egg	46	85	5	6	290	0
Hard-cooked, shell removed	1 egg	50	80	6	6	260	0
Poached	1 egg	50	80	6	6	260	0
Scrambled (milk added) in butter. Also omelet.	1 egg	64	95	6	7	310	0

FATS, OILS; RELATED PRODUCTS

		Grams	Cal.	Pro. (gm.)	Fat (gm.)	A (IU)	C (IU)
Butter:							
Regular (1 brick or 4 sticks per lb):							
Stick (½ cup)	1 stick	113	815	1	92	3,470	0
Tablespoon (about ⅛ stick).	1 tbsp.	14	100	trace	12	430	0

Pat (1 in square, ⅓ in high; 90 per lb).	1 pat	5	35	trace	4	150	0
Whipped (6 sticks or two 8-oz. containers per lb).							
Stick (½ cup)	1 stick	76	540	1	61	2,310	0
Tablespoon (about ⅛ stick).	1 tbsp	9	65	trace	8	290	0
Pat (1¼ in square, ⅓ in high; 120 per lb).	1 pat	4	25	trace	3	120	0
Fats, cooking (vegetable shortenings).	1 cup	200	1,770	0	200	—	0
	1 tbsp	13	110	0	13	—	0
Lard	1 cup	205	1,850	0	205	0	0
	1 tbsp	13	115	0	13	0	0
Margarine:							
Regular (1 brick or 4 sticks per lb):							
Stick (½ cup)	1 stick	113	815	1	92	[7]3,750	0
Tablespoon (about ⅛ stick)	1 tbsp	14	100	trace	12	[7]470	0
Pat (1 in square, ⅓ in high; 90 per lb).	1 pat	5	35	trace	4	[7]170	0

[7]Based on average Vitamin A content of fortified margarine. Federal specifications for fortified margarine require a minimum of 15,000 International Units (IU) of Vitamin A per pound.

FATS, OILS; RELATED PRODUCTS Cont

		Grams	Cal.	Pro. (gm.)	Fat (gm.)	A (IU)	C (IU)
Soft, two 8-oz containers per lb.	1 container	227	1,635	1	184	[7]7,500	0
	1 tbsp	14	100	trace	12	[7]470	0
Whipped (6 sticks per lb):							
Stick (½ cup)	1 stick	76	545	trace	61	[7]2,500	0
Tablespoon (about ⅛ stick)	1 tbsp	9	70	trace	8	[7]310	0
Oils, salad or cooking:							
Corn	1 cup	218	1,925	0	218	—	0
	1 tbsp	14	120	0	14	—	0
Olive	1 cup	216	1,910	0	216	—	0
	1 tbsp	14	120	0	14	—	0
Peanut	1 cup	216	1,910	0	216	—	0
	1 tbsp	14	120	0	14	—	0
Safflower	1 cup	218	1,925	0	218	—	0
	1 tbsp	14	120	0	14	—	0
Soybean oil, hydrogenated (partially hardened).	1 cup	218	1,925	0	218	—	0
	1 tbsp	14	120	0	14	—	0

Soybean—cottonseed oil blend, hydrogenated.	1 cup	218	1,925	0	218	—	0
	1 tbsp	14	120	0	14	—	0
Salad dressings:							
Commercial:							
Blue cheese:							
Regular	1 tbsp	15	75	1	8	30	trace
Low-calorie (5 Cal per tsp)	1 tbsp	16	10	trace	1	30	trace
French:							
Regular	1 tbsp	16	65	trace	6	—	—
Low-calorie (5 Cal per tsp)	1 tbsp	16	15	trace	1	—	—
Italian:							
Regular	1 tbsp	15	85	trace	9	—	—
Low-calorie (2 Cal. per tsp)	1 tbsp	15	10	trace	1	—	—
Mayonnaise	1 tbsp	14	100	trace	11	40	—
Mayonnaise type:							
Regular	1 tbsp	15	65	trace	6	30	—

[7]Based on average Vitamin A content of fortified margarine. Federal specifications for fortified margarine require a minimum of 15,000 International Units (IU) of Vitamin A per pound.

FATS, OILS; RELATED PRODUCTS *Cont.*

		Grams	Cal. (gm.)	Pro. (gm.)	Fat (gm.)	A (IU)	C (IU)
Low-calorie (8 Cal per tsp)	1 tbsp	16	20	trace	2	40	—
Tartar sauce, regular	1 tbsp	14	75	trace	8	30	trace
Thousand Island:							
Regular	1 tbsp	16	80	trace	8	50	trace
Low-calorie (10 Cal. per tsp)	1 tbsp	15	25	trace	2	50	trace
From home recipe:							
Cooked type	1 tbsp	16	25	1	2	80	trace

FISH, SHELLFISH, MEAT, POULTRY; RELATED PRODUCTS

		Grams	Cal. (gm.)	Pro. (gm.)	Fat (gm.)	A (IU)	C (IU)
Fish and shellfish:							
Bluefish, baked with butter or margarine.	3 oz	85	135	22	4	40	—
Clams:							
Raw, meat only	3 oz	85	65	11	1	90	8
Canned, solids and liquid	3 oz	85	45	7	1	—	—
Crabmeat (white or king), canned, not pressed down.	1 cup	135	135	24	3	—	—

Food	Measure						
Fish sticks, breaded, cooked, frozen (stick, 4 by 1 by ½ in).	1 fish stick or 1 oz	28	50	5	3	0	—
Haddock, breaded, fried[8]	3 oz	85	140	17	5	—	2
Ocean perch, breaded, fried[8]	1 fillet	85	195	16	11	—	—
Oysters, raw, meat only (13-19 medium Selects).	1 cup	240	160	20	4	740	—
Salmon: Broiled or Baked, with butter or margarine	1 lb	454	727	107.8	29.5	640	0
Salmon, pink, canned, solids and liquid.	3 oz	85	120	17	5	60	—
Salmon: Smoked	1 lb	454	798	98.0	42.2	0	0
	1 oz	28	50	6.1	2.6	0	0
Sardines[9], Atlantic, canned in oil, drained solids.	3 oz	85	175	20	9	190	—
Scallops, frozen, breaded, fried, reheated.	6 scallops	90	175	16	8	—	—
Shad, baked with butter or margarine, bacon.	3 oz	85	170	20	10	30	—
Shrimp: Canned meat	3 oz	85	100	21	1	50	—

[8] Dipped in egg, milk or water, and breadcrumbs; fried in vegetable shortening.

[9] If bones are discarded, value for calcium will be greatly reduced.

FISH, SHELLFISH, MEAT, POULTRY; RELATED PRODUCTS Cont.

	Grams	Cal. (gm.)	Pro. (gm.)	Fat (gm.)	A (IU)	C (IU)
French fried[10] .... 3 oz	85	190	17	9	—	—
Tuna, canned in oil, drained solids. .... 3 oz	85	170	24	7	70	—
Tuna salad[11] .... 1 cup	205	350	30	22	590	2
Meat and meat products:						
Bacon (20 slices per lb, raw), broiled or fried, crisp. .... 2 slices	15	85	4	8	0	—
Beef,[12] cooked:						
Cuts braised, simmered or pot roasted:						
Lean and fat (piece, 2½ by 2½ by ¾ in). .... 3 oz	85	245	23	16	30	—
Lean only .... 2.5 oz	72	140	22	5	10	—
Ground beef, broiled:						
Lean with 10% fat .... 3 oz or patty 3 by ⅝ in	85	185	23	10	20	—
Lean with 21% fat .... 2.9 oz or patty 3 by ⅝ in	82	235	20	17	30	—
Roast, oven cooked, no liquid added:						
Relatively fat, such as rib:						

Lean and fat (2 pieces, 4⅛ by 2¼ by ¼ in).	3 oz	85	375	17	33	70	—
Lean only from	1.8 oz	51	125	14	7	10	—
Relatively lean, such as heel of round:							
Lean and fat (2 pieces, 4⅛ by 2¼ by ¼ in).	3 oz	85	165	25	7	10	—
Lean only	2.8 oz	78	125	24	3	trace	—
Steak:							
Relatively fat—sirloin, broiled:							
Lean and fat (piece, 2½ by 2½ by ¾ in).	3 oz	85	330	20	27	50	—
Lean only	2.0 oz	56	115	18	4	10	—
Relatively lean—round, braised:							
Lean and fat (piece, 4⅛ by 2¼ by ½ in).	3 oz	85	220	24	13	20	—
Lean only	2.4 oz	68	130	21	4	10	—
Beef, canned:							

[10] Dipped in egg, breadcrumbs, and flour or batter.
[11] Prepared with tuna, celery, salad dressing (mayonnaise type), pickle, onion, and egg.
[12] Outer layer of fat on the cut was removed to within approximately ½ in of the lean. Deposits of fat within the cut were not removed.

FISH, SHELLFISH, MEAT, POULTRY; RELATED PRODUCTS Cont.

		Grams	Cal.	Pro. (gm.)	Fat (gm.)	A (IU)	C (IU)
Corned beef	3 oz	85	185	22	10	—	—
Corned beef hash	1 cup	220	400	19	25	—	—
Beef, dried, chipped	2½-oz jar	71	145	24	4	—	0
Beef and vegetable stew	1 cup	245	220	16	11	2,400	17
Beef potpie (home recipe), baked[13] (piece, ⅓ of 9-in diam. pie).	1 piece	210	515	21	30	1,720	6
Chili con carne with beans, canned.	1 cup	255	340	19	16	150	—
Chop suey with beef and pork (home recipe).	1 cup	250	300	26	17	600	33
Heart, beef, lean, braised	3 oz	85	160	27	5	20	1
Lamb, cooked:							
Chop, rib (cut 3 per lb with bone), broiled:							
Lean and fat	3.1 oz	89	360	18	32	—	—
Lean only	2 oz	57	120	16	6	—	—
Leg, roasted:							
Lean and fat (2 pieces, 4⅛ by 2¼ by ¼ in)	3 oz	85	235	22	16	—	—

Lean only	2.5 oz	71	130	20	5	—	—
Shoulder, roasted:							
Lean and fat (3 pieces, 2½ by 2½ by ¼ in)	3 oz	85	285	18	23	—	—
Lean only	2.3 oz	64	130	17	6	—	—
Liver, beef, fried[14] (slice, 6½ by 2⅜ by ⅜ in)	3 oz	85	195	22	9	[15]45,390	23
Pork, cured, cooked:							
Ham, light cure, lean and fat, roasted (2 pieces, 4⅛ by 2¼ by ¼ in)[16]	3 oz	85	245	18	19	0	—
Luncheon meat:							
Boiled ham, slice (8 per 8-oz pkg.)	1 oz	28	65	5	5	0	—
Canned, spiced or unspiced:							
Slice, approx. 3 by 2 by ½ in.	1 slice	60	175	9	15	0	—

[13]Crust made with vegetable shortening and enriched flour.
[14]Regular-type margarine used.
[15]Value varies widely.
[16]About one-fourth of the outer layer of fat on the cut was removed. Deposits of fat within the cut were not removed.

FISH, SHELLFISH, MEAT, POULTRY; RELATED PRODUCTS *Cont.*

	Grams	Cal.	Pro. (gm.)	Fat (gm.)	A (IU)	C (IU)
Pork, fresh, cooked:						
Chop, loin (cut 3 per lb with bone), broiled:						
Lean and fat ... 2.7 oz	78	305	19	25	0	—
Lean only ... 2 oz	56	150	17	9	0	—
Roast, oven cooked, no liquid added:						
Lean and fat (piece, 2½ by 2½ by ¾ in). ... 3 oz	85	310	21	24	0	—
Lean only ... 2.4 oz	68	175	20	10	0	—
Shoulder cut, simmered:						
Lean and fat (3 pieces, 2½ by 2½ by ¼ in). ... 3 oz	85	320	20	26	0	—
Lean only ... 2.2 oz	63	135	18	6	0	—
Sausages (see also Luncheon meat):						
Bologna, slice (8 per 8-oz pkg.). ... 1 slice	28	85	3	8	—	—
Braunschweiger, slice (6 per 6-oz pkg.). ... 1 slice	28	90	4	8	1,850	—

Food	Measure					
Brown and serve (10-11 per 8-oz pkg.), browned.	1 link	17	70	3	6	—
Deviled ham, canned	1 tbsp	13	45	2	4	0
Frankfurter (8 per 1-lb pkg.), cooked (reheated).	1 frankfurter	56	170	7	15	—
Meat, potted (beef, chicken, turkey), canned.	1 tbsp	13	30	2	2	—
Pork link (16 per 1-lb. pkg.), cooked.	1 link	13	60	2	6	0
Salami:						
Dry type, slice (12 per 4-oz pkg.).	1 slice	10	45	2	4	—
Cooked type, slice (8 per 8-oz pkg.).	1 slice	28	90	5	7	—
Vienna sausage (7 per 1-oz can).	1 sausage	16	40	2	3	—
Veal, medium fat, cooked, bone removed:						
Cutlet (4⅛ by 2¼ by ½ in), braised or broiled.	3 oz	85	185	23	9	—
Rib (2 pieces, 4⅛ by 2¼ by ¼ in), roasted.	3 oz	85	230	23	14	—

FISH, SHELLFISH, MEAT, POULTRY; RELATED PRODUCTS *Cont.*

		Grams (gm.)	Cal.	Pro. (gm.)	Fat (gm.)	A (IU)	C (IU)
Poultry and poultry products:							
Chicken, cooked:							
Breast, fried, bones removed, ½ breast (3.3 oz with bones).	2.8 oz	79	160	26	5	70	—
Drumstick, fried, bones removed (2 oz with bones).	1.3 oz	38	90	12	4	50	—
Half broiler, broiled, bones removed (10.4 oz with bones).	6.2 oz	176	240	42	7	160	—
Chicken, canned, boneless	3 oz	85	170	18	10	200	3
Chicken a la king, cooked (home recipe).	1 cup	245	470	27	34	1,130	12
Chicken and noodles, cooked (home recipe).	1 cup	240	365	22	8	430	trace
Chicken chow mein:							
Canned	1 cup	250	95	7	trace	150	13
From home recipe	1 cup	250	255	31	10	280	10
Chicken potpie (home recipe), baked, piece (⅓ or 9-in diam. pie).	1 piece	232	545	23	31	3,090	5

Turkey, roasted, flesh without skin:

Food	Measure	g	cal					
Dark meat, piece, 2½ by 1⅝ by ¼ in.	4 pieces	85	175	26	7	—	—	—
Light meat, piece, 4 by 2 by ¼ in.	2 pieces	85	150	28	3	—	—	—
Light and dark meat:								
Chopped or diced	1 cup	140	265	44	9		—	—
Pieces (1 slice white meat, 4 by 2 by ¼ in with 2 slices dark meat, 2½ by 1⅝ by ¼ in).	3 pieces	85	160	27	5		—	—

FRUITS AND FRUIT PRODUCTS

Apples, raw, unpeeled, without cores:

Food	Measure	g	cal					
2 ¾-in diam. (about 3 per lb with cores).	1 apple	138	80	trace	1	120	6
3 ¼ in diam. (about 2 per lb with cores).	1 apple	212	125	trace	1	190	8
Applejuice,[17] bottled or canned	1 cup	248	120	trace	trace	—	2

[17] Applies to product without added ascorbic acid. For value of product with added ascorbic acid, refer to label.

FRUIT AND FRUIT PRODUCTS Cont.

		Grams	Cal. (gm.)	Pro. (gm.)	Fat (gm.)	A (IU)	C (IU)
Applesauce, canned:							
Sweetened	1 cup	255	230	1	trace	100	3
Unsweetened	1 cup	244	100	trace	trace	100	2
Apricots:							
Raw, without pits (about 12 per lb with pits).	3 apricots	107	55	1	trace	2,890	11
Canned in heavy sirup (halves and sirup).	1 cup	258	220	2	trace	4,490	10
Dried:							
Uncooked (28 large or 37 medium halves per cup).	1 cup	130	340	7	1	14,170	16
Cooked, unsweetened, fruit and liquid.	1 cup	250	215	4	1	7,500	8
Apricot nectar, canned	1 cup	251	145	1	trace	2,380	36
Avocados, raw, whole, without skins and seeds:							
California, mid- and late-winter (with skin and seed, 3⅛-in diam.; wt., 10 oz).	1 avocado	216	370	5	37	630	30
Florida, late summer and fall	1 avocado	304	390	4	33	880	43

(with skin and seed, 3⅝-in diam.; wt., 1 lb).							
Banana without peel (about 2.6 per lb with peel).	1 banana	119	100	1	trace	230	12
Banana flakes	1 tbsp	6	20	trace	trace	50	trace
Blackberries, raw	1 cup	144	85	2	1	290	30
Blueberries, raw	1 cup	145	90	1	1	150	20
Cantaloupe. See Muskmelons							
Cherries:							
Sour (tart), red, pitted, canned, water pack.	1 cup	244	105	2	trace	1,660	12
Sweet, raw, without pits and stems.	10 cherries	68	45	1	trace	70	7
Cranberry juice cocktail, bottled, sweetened.	1 cup	253	165	trace	trace	trace	[18]81
Cranberry sauce, sweetened, canned, strained.	1 cup	277	405	trace	1	60	6
Dates:							
Whole, without pits	10 dates	80	220	2	trace	40	0
Chopped	1 cup	178	490	4	1	90	0
Fruit cocktail, canned, in heavy sirup.	1 cup	255	195	1	trace	360	5

[18]Based on product with label claim of 100% of U.S. RDA in 6 fl oz.

FRUIT AND FRUIT PRODUCTS Cont.

	Grams	Cal. (gm.)	Pro. (gm.)	Fat (gm.)	A (IU)	C (IU)
Grapefruit:						
Raw, medium, 3¾-in diam. (about 1 lb 1 oz):						
Pink or red ½ grapefruit with peel[19]	241	50	1	trace	540	44
White ½ grapefruit with peel[19]	241	45	1	trace	10	44
Canned, sections with sirup 1 cup	254	180	2	trace	30	76
Grapefruit juice:						
Raw, pink, red, or white 1 cup	246	95	1	trace	(20)	93
Canned, white:						
Unsweetened 1 cup	247	100	1	trace	20	84
Sweetened 1 cup	250	135	1	trace	30	78
Frozen, concentrate, unsweetened:						
Undiluted, 6-fl oz can 1 can	207	300	4	1	60	286
Diluted with 3 parts water 1 cup by volume.	247	100	1	trace	20	96
Dehydrated crystals, prepared 1 cup with water (1 lb yields about 1 gal).	247	100	1	trace	20	91
Grapes, European type (adherent skin), raw:						

Food	Measure	Grams	Food energy (calories)	Protein (g)	Fat (g)	Vitamin A (I.U.)	Ascorbic acid (mg)
Thompson Seedless	10 grapes	50	35	trace	trace	50	2
Tokay and Emperor, seeded types	10 grapes[21]	60	40	trace	trace	60	2
Grapejuice:							
Canned or bottled	1 cup	253	165	1	1	—[17]trace	trace
Frozen concentrate, sweetened:							
Undiluted, 6-fl oz can	1 can	216	395	1	1	40	[22]32
Diluted with 3 parts water by volume.	1 cup	250	135	1	1	10	[22]10
Grape drink, canned	1 cup	250	135	trace	trace	—	([23])
Lemon, raw, size 165, without peel and seeds (about 4 per lb with peels and seeds).	1 lemon	74	20	1	trace	10	39
Lemon juice:							
Raw	1 cup	244	60	1	trace	50	112
Canned, or bottled, unsweetened	1 cup	244	55	1	trace	50	102

[19] Weight includes peel and membranes between sections.

[20] For white-fleshed varieties, value is about 20 International Units (IU) per cup; for red-fleshed varieties, 1,080 IU.

[21] Weight includes seeds. Without seeds, weight of the edible portion is 57 g.

[22] Applies to product without added ascorbic acid. 36 or 40 for 1 cup of diluted juice.

[23] For products with added thiamin and riboflavin but without added ascorbic acid, values in milligrams would be 0.60 for thiamin, 0.80 for riboflavin, and trace for ascorbic acid. For products with only ascorbic acid added, value varies with the brand. Consult the label.

FRUIT AND FRUIT PRODUCTS *Cont.*

		Grams	Cal. (gm.)	Pro. (gm.)	Fat (gm.)	A (IU)	C (IU)
Frozen, single strength, unsweetened, 6-fl oz can.	1 can	183	40	1	trace	40	81
Lemonade concentrate, frozen:							
Undiluted, 6-fl oz can	1 can	219	425	trace	trace	40	66
Diluted with 4⅓ parts water by volume.	1 cup	248	105	trace	trace	10	17
Limeade concentrate, frozen:							
Undiluted, 6-fl oz can	1 can	218	410	trace	trace	trace	26
Diluted with 4⅓ parts water by volume.	1 cup	247	100	trace	trace	trace	6
Limejuice:							
Raw	1 cup	246	65	1	trace	20	79
Canned, unsweetened	1 cup	246	65	1	trace	20	52
Mango	1 fruit	300	152	1.6	.9	437	81
Muskmelons, raw, with rind, without seed cavity:							
Cantaloupe, orange-fleshed (with rind and seed cavity, 5-in diam., 2⅓ lb).	½ melon with rind	477	80	2	trace	9,240	90
Honeydew (with rind and seed cavity, 6½-in diam., 5¼ lb).	1/10 melon with rind	226	50	1	trace	60	34

Oranges, all commercial varieties, raw:							
Whole, 2⅝-in diam., without peel and seeds (about 2½ per lb with peel and seeds).	1 orange	131	65	1	trace	260	66
Sections without membranes	1 cup	180	90	2	trace	360	90
Orange juice:							
Raw, all varieties	1 cup	248	110	2	trace	500	124
Canned, unsweetened	1 cup	249	120	2	trace	500	100
Frozen concentrate:							
Undiluted, 6-fl oz can	1 can	213	360	5	trace	1,620	360
Diluted with 3 parts water by volume.	1 cup	249	120	2	trace	540	120
Dehydrated crystals, prepared with water (1 lb yields about 1 gal).	1 cup	248	115	1	trace	500	109
Orange and grapefruit juice:							
Frozen concentrate:							
Undiluted, 6-fl oz can	1 can	210	330	4	1	800	302
Diluted with 3 parts water by volume.	1 cup	248	110	1	trace	270	102
Papayas, raw, ½-in cubes	1 cup	140	55	1	trace	2,450	78

FRUIT AND FRUIT PRODUCTS *Cont.*

		Grams	Cal. (gm.)	Pro. (gm.)	Fat (gm.)	A (IU)	C (IU)
Peaches:							
Raw:							
Whole, 2½-in diam., peeled, pitted (about 4 per lb with peels and pits).	1 peach	100	40	1	trace	1,330	7
Sliced	1 cup	170	65	1	trace	2,260	12
Canned, yellow-fleshed, solids and liquid (halves or slices):							
Sirup pack	1 cup	256	200	1	trace	1,100	8
Water pack	1 cup	244	75	1	trace	1,100	7
Dried:							
Uncooked	1 cup	160	420	5	1	6,240	29
Cooked, unsweetened, halves and juice.	1 cup	250	205	3	1	3,050	5
Frozen, sliced, sweetened:							
10-oz container	1 container	284	250	1	trace	1,850	116
Cup	1 cup	250	220	1	trace	1,630	103
Pears:							
Raw, with skin, cored:							
Bartlett, 2½-in diam. (about	1 pear	164	100	1	1	30	7

2½ per lb with cores and stems).							
Bosc, 2½-in diam. (about 3 per lb with cores and stems).	1 pear	141	85	1	1	30	6
D'Anjou, 3-in diam. (about 2 per lb with cores and stems).	1 pear	200	120	1	1	40	8
Canned, solids and liquid, sirup pack, heavy (halves or slices).	1 cup	255	195	1	1	10	3
Pineapple:							
Raw, diced	1 cup	155	80	trace	1	110	26
Canned, heavy sirup pack, solids and liquid:							
Crushed, chunks, tidbits	1 cup	255	190	1	trace	130	18
Slices and liquid:							
Large	1 slice; 2¼ tbsp liquid.	105	80	trace	trace	50	7
Medium	1 slice; 1¼ tbsp liquid.	58	45	trace	trace	30	4
Pineapple juice, unsweetened, canned.	1 cup	250	140	1	trace	130	80

FRUIT AND FRUIT PRODUCTS Cont.

		Grams	Cal.	Pro. (gm.)	Fat (gm.)	A (IU)	C (IU)
Plums:							
Raw, without pits:							
Japanese and hybrid (2⅛-in diam., about 6½ per lb with pits).	1 plum	66	30	trace	trace	160	4
Prune-type (1½-in diam., about 15 per lb with pits).	1 plum	28	20	trace	trace	80	1
Canned, heavy sirup pack (Italian prunes), with pits and liquid:							
Cup	1 cup	272	215	1	trace	3,130	5
Portion	3 plums; 2¾ tbsp liquid	140	110	1	trace	1,610	3
Prunes, dried, "softenized," with pits:							
Uncooked	4 extra large or 5 large prunes	49	110	1	trace	690	1
Cooked, unsweetened, all sizes, fruit and liquid.	1 cup	250	255	2	1	1,590	2
Prune juice, canned or bottled	1 cup	256	195	1	trace	—	5
Raisins, seedless:							
Cup, not pressed down	1 cup	145	420	4	trace	30	1

Packet, ½ oz. (1½ tbsp)	1 packet	14	40	trace	trace	trace	trace
Raspberries, red:							
Raw, capped, whole	1 cup	123	70	1	1	160	31
Frozen, sweetened, 10-oz container	1 container	284	280	2	1	200	60
Rhubarb, cooked, added sugar:							
From raw	1 cup	270	380	1	trace	220	16
From frozen, sweetened	1 cup	270	385	1	1	190	16
Strawberries:							
Raw, whole berries, capped	1 cup	149	55	1	1	90	88
Frozen, sweetened:							
Sliced, 10-oz container	1 container	284	310	1	1	90	151
Whole, 1-lb container (about 1¾ cups)	1 container	454	415	2	1	140	249
Tangerine, raw, 2⅜-in diam., size 176, without peel (about 4 per lb with peels and seeds).	1 tangerine	86	40	1	trace	360	27
Tangerine juice, canned, sweetened.	1 cup	249	125	1	trace	1,040	54
Watermelon, raw, 4 by 8 in wedge with rind and seeds (1/16 of 32 ⅔-lb melon, 10 by 16 in).	1 wedge with rind and seeds	926	110	2	1	2,510	30

GRAIN PRODUCTS

		Grams	Cal. (gm.)	Pro. (gm.)	Fat (gm.)	A (IU)	C (IU)
Bagel, 3-in diam.:							
Egg	1 bagel	55	165	6	2	30	0
Water	1 bagel	55	165	6	1	0	0
Barley, pearled, light, uncooked	1 cup	200	700	16	2	0	0
Biscuits, baking powder, 2-in diam. (enriched flour, vegetable shortening):							
From home recipe	1 biscuit	28	105	2	5	trace	trace
From mix	1 biscuit	28	90	2	3	trace	trace
Breadcrumbs (enriched):							
Dry, grated	1 cup	100	390	13	5	trace	trace
Soft. See White bread.							
Breads:							
Boston brown bread, canned slice, 3¼ by ½ in.	1 slice	45	95	2	1	0	0
Cracked-wheat bread (¾ enriched wheat flour, ¼ cracked wheat):							
Loaf, 1 lb	1 loaf	454	1,195	39	10	trace	trace

Food	Measure						
Slice (18 per loaf)	1 slice	25	65	2	1	trace	trace
French or vienna bread, enriched:							
Loaf, 1 lb	1 loaf	454	1,315	41	14	trace	trace
Slice:							
French (5 by 2½ by 1 in)	1 slice	35	100	3	1	trace	trace
Vienna (4¾ by 4 by ½ in)	1 slice	25	75	2	1	trace	trace
Italian bread, enriched:							
Loaf, 1 lb	1 loaf	454	1,250	41	4	0	0
Slice, 4½ by 3¼ by ¾ in.	1 slice	30	85	3	trace	0	0
Raisin bread, enriched:							
Loaf, 1 lb	1 loaf	454	1,190	30	13	trace	trace
Slice (18 per loaf)	1 slice	25	65	2	1	trace	trace
Rye Bread:							
American, light (⅔ enriched wheat flour, ⅓ rye flour):							
Loaf, 1 lb	1 loaf	454	1,100	41	5	0	0
Slice (4¾ by 3¾ by 7/16 in)	1 slice	25	60	2	trace	0	0
Pumpernickel (⅔ rye flour, ⅓ enriched wheat flour):							
Loaf, 1 lb	1 loaf	454	1,115	41	5	0	0

GRAIN PRODUCTS Cont.

		Grams	Cal.	Pro. (gm.)	Fat (gm.)	A (IU)	C (IU)
Slice (5 by 4 by ⅜ in)	1 slice	32	80	3	trace	0	0
White bread, enriched:[24]							
Soft-crumb type:							
Loaf, 1 lb	1 loaf	454	1,225	39	15	trace	trace
Slice (18 per loaf)	1 slice	25	70	2	1	trace	trace
Slice, toasted	1 slice	22	70	2	1	trace	trace
Slice (22 per loaf)	1 slice	20	55	2	1	trace	trace
Slice, toasted	1 slice	17	55	2	1	trace	trace
Loaf, 1½ lb	1 loaf	680	1,835	59	22	trace	trace
Slice (24 per loaf)	1 slice	28	75	2	1	trace	trace
Slice, toasted	1 slice	24	75	2	1	trace	trace
Slice (28 per loaf)	1 slice	24	65	2	1	trace	trace
Slice, toasted	1 slice	21	65	2	1	trace	trace
Cubes	1 cup	30	80	3	1	trace	trace
Crumbs	1 cup	45	120	4	1	trace	trace
Firm-crumb type:							
Loaf, 1 lb	1 loaf	454	1,245	41	17	trace	trace
Slice (20 per loaf)	1 slice	23	65	2	1	trace	trace
Slice, toasted	1 slice	20	65	2	1	trace	trace
Loaf, 2 lb	1 loaf	907	2,495	82	34	trace	trace

Slice (34 per loaf)	1 slice	27	75	2	1	trace	trace
Slice, toasted	1 slice	23	75	2	1	trace	trace
Whole-wheat bread:							
Soft-crumb type:[24]							
Loaf, 1 lb	1 loaf	454	1,095	41	12	trace	trace
Slice (16 per loaf)	1 slice	28	65	3	1	trace	trace
Slice, toasted	1 slice	24	65	3	1	trace	trace
Firm-crumb type:[24]							
Loaf, 1 lb	1 loaf	454	1,100	48	14	trace	trace
Slice (18 per loaf)	1 slice	25	60	3	1	trace	trace
Slice, toasted	1 slice	21	60	3	1	trace	trace
Breakfast cereals:							
Hot type, cooked:							
Corn (hominy) grits, degermed:							
Enriched	1 cup	245	125	3	trace	[25]trace	0
Unenriched	1 cup	245	125	3	trace	[25]trace	0
Farina, quick-cooking, enriched.	1 cup	245	105	3	trace	0	0
Oatmeal or rolled oats	1 cup	240	130	5	2	0	0
Wheat, rolled	1 cup	240	180	5	1	0	0

[24]Made with vegetable shortening.
[25]Applies to white varieties. For yellow varieties, value is 150 International Units (IU)

GRAIN PRODUCTS Cont.

	Grams	Cal. (gm.)	Pro. (gm.)	Fat (gm.)	A (IU)	C (IU)
Wheat, whole-meal 1 cup	245	110	4	1	0	0
Ready-to-eat:						
Bran flakes (40% bran), added sugar, salt, iron, vitamins. 1 cup	35	105	4	1	1,540	0
Bran flakes with raisins, added sugar, salt, iron, vitamins. 1 cup	50	145	4	1	[26]2,200	0
Corn flakes:						
Plain, added sugar, salt, iron, vitamins. 1 cup	25	95	2	trace	([27])	[28]13
Sugar-coated, added salt, iron, vitamins. 1 cup	40	155	2	trace	1,760	[28]21
Corn, oat flour, puffed, added sugar, salt, iron, vitamins. 1 cup	20	80	2	1	880	11
Corn, shredded, added sugar, salt, iron, thiamin, niacin. 1 cup	25	95	2	trace	0	13
Oats, puffed, added sugar, salt, minerals, vitamins. 1 cup	25	100	3	1	1,100	13

Rice, puffed:							
Plain, added iron, thiamin, niacin.	1 cup	15	60	1	trace	0	0
Presweetened, added salt, iron, vitamins.	1 cup	28	115	1	0	[28]1,240	[28]15
Wheat flakes, added sugar, salt, iron, vitamins.	1 cup	30	105	3	trace	1,320	16
Wheat, puffed:							
Plain, added iron, thiamin, niacin.	1 cup	15	55	2	trace	0	0
Presweetened, added salt, iron, vitamins.	1 cup	38	140	3	trace	1,680	[28]20
Wheat, shredded, plain	1 oblong biscuit or ½ cup spoon-size biscuits.	25	90	2	1	0	0
Wheat germ, without salt and sugar, toasted.	1 tbsp	6	25	2	1	10	1
Buckwheat flour, light, sifted	1 cup	98	340	6	1	0	0
Bulgur, canned, seasoned	1 cup	135	245	8	4	0	0
Bulgur, dry Raw	1 cup	175	628	15.2	2.5	0	0

[26]Applies to product with added nutrient. Without added nutrient, value is trace.

[27]Value varies with the brand. Consult the label.

[28]Applies to product with added nutrient. Without added nutrient, value is trace.

GRAIN PRODUCTS Cont.

		Grams	Cal.	Pro. (gm.)	Fat (gm.)	A (IU)	C (IU)
Cake icings. See Sugars and Sweets							
Cakes made from cake mixes with enriched flour:[29]							
Angel food:							
Whole cake (9¾-in diam. tube cake).	1 cake	635	1,645	36	1	0	0
Piece, 1/12 of cake	1 piece	53	135	3	trace	0	0
Coffeecake:							
Whole cake (7¾ by 5⅝ by 1¼ in).	1 cake	430	1,385	27	41	690	1
Piece, ⅙ of cake	1 piece	72	230	5	7	120	trace
Cupcakes, made with egg, milk, 2½-in diam.:							
Without icing	1 cupcake	25	90	1	3	40	trace
With chocolate icing	1 cupcake	36	130	2	5	60	trace
Devil's food with chocolate icing:							
Whole, 2 layer cake (8- or 9-in diam.).	1 cake	1,107	3,755	49	136	1,660	1

Piece, 1/16 of cake	1 piece	69	235	3	8	100	trace
Cupcake, 2½-in diam.	1 cupcake	35	120	2	4	50	trace
Gingerbread:							
Whole cake (8-in square)	1 cake	570	1,575	18	39	trace	trace
Piece, 1/9 of cake	1 piece	63	175	2	4	trace	trace
White, 2 layer with chocolate icing;							
Whole cake (8- or 9-in diam.)	1 cake	1,140	4,000	44	122	680	2
Piece, 1/16 of cake	1 piece	71	250	3	8	40	trace
Yellow, 2 layer with chocolate icing;							
Whole cake (8- or 9-in diam.)	1 cake	1,108	3,735	45	125	1,550	2
Piece, 1/16 of cake	1 piece	69	235	3	8	100	trace
Cakes made from home recipes using enriched flour:[30]							
Boston cream pie with custard filling:							
Whole cake (8-in diam.)	1 cake	825	2,490	41	78	1,730	2
Piece, 1/12 of cake	1 piece	69	210	3	6	140	trace

[29]Excepting angel food cake, cakes were made from mixes containing vegetable shortening; icings, with butter.

[30]Excepting spongecake, vegetable shortening used for cake portion; butter, for icing. If butter or margarine used for cake portion, Vitamin A values would be higher.

GRAIN PRODUCTS *Cont.*

		Grams	Cal.	Pro. (gm.)	Fat (gm.)	A (IU)	C (IU)
Fruitcake, dark:							
Loaf, 1-lb (7½ by 2 by 1½ in).	1 loaf	454	1,720	22	69	540	2
Slice, 1/30 of loaf.	1 slice	15	55	1	2	20	trace
Plain, sheet cake:							
Without icing:							
Whole cake (9-in square)	1 cake	777	2,830	35	108	1,320	2
Piece, 1/9 of cake	1 piece	86	315	4	12	150	trace
With uncooked white icing:							
Whole cake (9-in square)	1 cake	1,096	4,020	37	129	2,190	2
Piece, 1/9 of cake	1 piece	121	445	4	14	240	trace
Pound:[31]							
Loaf, 8½ by 3½ by 3¼ in.	1 loaf	565	2,725	31	170	1,410	0
Slice, 1/17 of loaf	1 slice	33	160	2	10	80	0
Spongecake:							
Whole cake (9¾-in diam. tube cake).	1 cake	790	2,345	60	45	3,560	trace
Piece, 1/12 of cake	1 piece	66	195	5	4	300	trace
Cookies made with enriched flour:[32][33]							

Brownies with nuts:						
Home-prepared, 1¾ by 1¾ by ⅞ in:						
From home recipe	1 brownie	20	95	1	6	40	trace
From commercial recipe	1 brownie	20	85	1	4	20	trace
Frozen, with chocolate icing,[34] 1½ by 1¾ by ⅞ in.	1 brownie	25	105	1	5	50	trace
Chocolate chip:						
Commercial, 2¼-in diam., ⅜ in thick.	4 cookies	42	200	2	9	50	trace
From home recipe, 2⅓-in diam.	4 cookies	40	205	2	12	40	trace
Fig bars, square (1⅝ by 1⅝ by ⅜ in) or rectangular (1½ by 1¾ by ½ in).	4 cookies	56	200	2	3	60	trace
Gingersnaps, 2-in diam., ¼ in thick.	4 cookies	28	90	2	2	20	0
Macaroons, 2¾-in diam., ¼ in thick.	2 cookies	38	180	2	9	0	0

[31]Equal weights of flour, sugar, eggs, and vegetable shortening.
[32]Products are commercial unless otherwise specified.
[33]Made with enriched flour and vegetable shortening except for macaroons which do not contain flour or shortening.
[34]Icing made with butter.

GRAIN PRODUCTS *Cont.*

		Grams	Cal.	Pro. (gm.)	Fat (gm.)	A (IU)	C (IU)
Oatmeal with raisins, 2⅝-in diam., ¼ in thick.	4 cookies	52	235	3	8	30	trace
Plain, prepared from commercial chilled dough, 2½-in diam., ¼ in thick.	4 cookies	48	240	2	12	30	0
Sandwich type (chocolate or vanilla), 1¾-in diam., ⅜ in thick.	4 cookies	40	200	2	9	0	0
Vanilla wafers, 1¾-in diam., ¼ in thick.	10 cookies	40	185	2	6	50	0
Cornmeal:							
Whole-ground, unbolted, dry form.	1 cup	122	435	11	5	[36]620	0
Bolted (nearly whole-grain), dry form.	1 cup	122	440	11	4	[36]590	0
Degermed, enriched:							
Dry form	1 cup	138	500	11	2	[36]610	0
Cooked	1 cup	240	120	3	trace	[36]140	0
Degermed, unenriched:							
Dry form	1 cup	138	500	11	2	[36]610	0
Cooked	1 cup	240	120	3	trace	[36]140	0

Crackers:[35]							
Graham, plain, 2½-in square	2 crackers	14	55	1	1		0
Rye wafers, whole-grain, 1⅞ by 3½ in.	2 wafers	13	45	2	trace		0
Saltines, made with enriched flour.	4 crackers or 1 packet	11	50	1	1		0
Danish pastry (enriched flour), plain without fruit or nuts:[37]							
Packaged ring, 12 oz	1 ring	340	1,435	25	80	1,050	trace
Round piece, about 4¼-in diam. by 1 in.	1 pastry	65	275	5	15	200	trace
Ounce	1 oz	28	120	2	7	90	trace
Doughnuts, made with enriched flour:[38]							
Cake type, plain, 2½-in diam., 1 in high.	1 doughnut	25	100	1	5	20	trace
Yeast-leavened, glazed, 3¾-in diam., 1¼ in. high.	1 doughnut	50	205	3	11	25	0

[35]Made with vegetable shortening.
[36]Applies to yellow varieties; white varieties contain only a trace.
[37]Contains vegetable shortening and butter.
[38]Made with corn oil.

GRAIN PRODUCTS Cont.

	Grams	Cal. (gm.)	Pro. (gm.)	Fat (gm.)	A (IU)	C (IU)
Macaroni, enriched, cooked (cut lengths, elbows, shells):						
Firm stage (hot) .... 1 cup	130	190	7	1	0	0
Tender stage:						
Cold macaroni ...... 1 cup	105	115	4	trace	0	0
Hot macaroni ...... 1 cup	140	155	5	1	0	0
Macaroni (enriched) and cheese:						
Canned[38] ...... 1 cup	240	230	9	10	260	trace
From home recipe (served hot)[39] ...... 1 cup	200	430	17	22	860	trace
Muffins made with enriched flour:[39]						
From home recipe:						
Blueberry, 2⅜-in diam., 1½ in high. ...... 1 muffin	40	110	3	4	90	trace
Bran ...... 1 muffin	40	105	3	4	90	trace
Corn (enriched degermed cornmeal and flour), 2⅜-in diam., 1½ in high. ...... 1 muffin	40	125	3	4	120	trace

Plain, 3-in diam., 1½ in high.	1 muffin	40	120	3	4	40	trace
From mix, egg, milk:							
Corn, 2⅜-in diam., 1½ in high.[41]	1 muffin	40	130	3	4	[40]100	trace
Noodles (egg noodles), enriched, cooked.	1 cup	160	200	7	2	110	0
Noodles, chow mein, canned.	1 cup	45	220	6	11	—	—
Pancakes (4-in diam.):							
Buckwheat, made from mix (with buckwheat and enriched flours), egg and milk added.	1 cake	27	55	2	2	60	trace
Plain:							
Made from home recipe using enriched flour.	1 cake	27	60	2	2	30	trace
Made from mix with enriched flour, egg and milk added.	1 cake	27	60	2	2	70	trace
Pies, piecrust made with enriched flour, vegetable shortening (9-in diam.):							

[39] Made with regular margarine.
[40] Applies to product made with yellow cornmeal.
[41] Made with enriched degermed cornmeal and enriched flour.

GRAIN PRODUCTS *Cont.*

		Grams	Cal.	Pro. (gm.)	Fat (gm.)	A (IU)	C (IU)
Apple:							
Whole	1 pie	945	2,420	21	105	280	9
Sector, ⅐ of pie	1 sector	135	345	3	15	40	2
Banana cream:							
Whole	1 pie	910	2,010	41	85	2,280	9
Sector, ⅐ of pie	1 sector	130	285	6	12	330	1
Blueberry:							
Whole	1 pie	945	2,285	23	102	280	28
Sector, ⅐ of pie	1 sector	135	325	3	15	40	4
Cherry:							
Whole	1 pie	945	2,465	25	107	4,160	trace
Sector, ⅐ of pie	1 sector	135	350	4	15	590	trace
Custard:							
Whole	1 pie	910	1,985	56	101	2,090	0
Sector, ⅐ of pie	1 sector	130	285	8	14	300	0
Lemon meringue:							
Whole	1 pie	840	2,140	31	86	1,430	25
Sector, ⅐ of pie	1 sector	120	305	4	12	200	4
Mince:							
Whole	1 pie	945	2,560	24	109	20	9
Sector, ⅐ of pie	1 sector	135	365	3	16	trace	1

Peach:							
Whole	1 pie	945	2,410	24	101	6,900	28
Sector, 1/6 of pie	1 sector	135	345	3	14	990	4
Pecan:							
Whole	1 pie	825	3,450	42	189	1,320	trace
Sector, 1/6 of pie	1 sector	118	495	6	27	190	trace
Pumpkin:							
Whole	1 pie	910	1,920	36	102	22,480	trace
Sector, 1/6 of pie	1 sector	130	275	5	15	3,210	trace
Piecrust (home recipe) made with enriched flour and vegetable shortening, baked.	1 pie shell, 9-in diam.	180	900	11	60	0	0
Piecrust mix with enriched flour and vegetable shortening, 10-oz pkg. prepared and baked.	Piecrust for 2-crust pie, 9-in diam.	320	1,485	20	93	0	0
Pizza (cheese) baked, 4¾-in sector; ⅛ of 12-in diam. pie.	1 sector	60	145	6	4	230	4
Popcorn, popped:							
Plain, large kernel	1 cup	6	25	1	trace	—	0
With oil (coconut) and salt added, large kernel.	1 cup	9	40	1	2	—	0
Sugar coated	1 cup	35	135	2	1	—	0

GRAIN PRODUCTS *Cont.*

		Grams	Cal. (gm.)	Pro. (gm.)	Fat (gm.)	A (IU)	C (IU)
Pretzels, made with enriched flour:							
Dutch, twisted, 2¾ by 2⅝ in.	1 pretzel	16	60	2	1	0	0
Thin, twisted, 3¼ by 2¼ by ¼ in.	10 pretzels	60	235	6	3	0	0
Stick, 2¼ in long	10 pretzels	3	10	trace	trace	0	0
Rice:							
Brown							
Raw	1 cup	185	666	13.9	3.5	0	0
Rice, white, enriched:							
Instant, ready-to-serve, hot	1 cup	165	180	4	trace	0	0
Long grain:							
Raw	1 cup	185	670	12	1	0	0
Cooked, served hot	1 cup	205	225	4	trace	0	0
Parboiled:							
Raw	1 cup	185	685	14	1	0	0
Cooked, served hot	1 cup	175	185	4	trace	0	0
Rolls, enriched:							
Commercial:							
Brown-and-serve (12 per 12-oz pkg.), browned.	1 roll	26	85	2	2	trace	trace

Cloverleaf or pan, 2½-in diam., 2 in high.	1 roll	28	85	2	2	trace	trace
Frankfurter and hamburger (8 per 11½-oz pkg.).	1 roll	40	120	3	2	trace	trace
Hard, 3¾-in diam., 2 in high.	1 roll	50	155	5	2	trace	trace
Hoagie or submarine, 11½ by 3 by 2½ in.	1 roll	135	390	12	4	trace	trace
From home recipe:							
Cloverleaf, 2½-in diam., 2 in high.	1 roll	35	120	3	3	30	trace
Spaghetti, enriched, cooked:							
Firm stage, "al dente," served hot.	1 cup	130	190	7	1	0	0
Tender stage, served hot	1 cup	140	155	5	1	0	0
Spaghetti: Enriched Dry	8 ounces	227	838	28.4	2.7	0	0
Spaghetti: Whole Wheat Dry	8 ounces	227	840	100	8	0	0

GRAIN PRODUCTS Cont.

		Grams	Cal.	Pro. (gm.)	Fat (gm.)	A (IU)	C (IU)
Spaghetti (enriched) in tomato sauce with cheese:							
From home recipe	1 cup	250	260	9	9	1,080	13
Canned	1 cup	250	190	6	2	930	10
Spaghetti (enriched) with meat balls and tomato sauce:							
From home recipe	1 cup	248	330	19	12	1,590	22
Canned	1 cup	250	260	12	10	1,000	5
Toaster pastries	1 pastry	50	200	3	6	500	[42]
Waffles, made with enriched flour, 7-in diam.:							
From home recipe	1 waffle	75	210	7	7	250	trace
From mix, egg and milk added	1 waffle	75	205	7	8	170	trace
Wheat flours:							
All-purpose or family flour, enriched:							
Sifted, spooned	1 cup	115	420	12	1	0	0
Unsifted, spooned	1 cup	125	455	13	1	0	0
Cake or pastry flour, enriched, sifted, spooned.	1 cup	96	350	7	1	0	0

Self-rising, enriched, unsifted, spooned.	1 cup	125	440	12	1	0	0
Whole-wheat, from hard wheats, stirred.	1 cup	120	400	16	2	0	0

LEGUMES (DRY), NUTS, SEEDS; RELATED PRODUCTS

Almonds, shelled:							
Chopped (about 130 almonds)	1 cup	130	775	24	70	0	trace
Slivered, not pressed down (about 115 almonds).	1 cup	115	690	21	62	0	trace
Beans, dry:							
Common varieties as Great Northern, navy, and others:							
Cooked, drained:							
Great Northern	1 cup	180	210	14	1	1	0
Pea (navy)	1 cup	190	225	15	1	1	0
Canned, solids and liquid:							
White with—							
Frankfurters (sliced)	1 cup	255	365	19	18	330	trace
Pork and tomato sauce	1 cup	255	310	16	7	330	5
Pork and sweet sauce	1 cup	255	385	16	12	—	—
Red kidney	1 cup	255	230	15	1	10	—

[42]Value varies with the brand. Consult the label.

LEGUMES (DRY), NUTS, SEEDS; RELATED PRODUCTS *Cont.*

		Grams	Cal. (gm.)	Pro. (gm.)	Fat (gm.)	A (IU)	C (IU)
Lima, cooked, drained	1 cup	190	260	16	1	—	—
Blackeye peas, dry, cooked (with residual cooking liquid).	1 cup	250	190	13	1	30	—
Brazil nuts, shelled (6–8 large kernels).	1 oz	28	185	4	19	trace	—
Cashew nuts, roasted in oil	1 cup	140	785	24	64	140	—
Chickpeas:							
Raw	1 cup	240	367	22.3	18.5	430	trace
Dry							
Coconut meat, fresh:							
Piece, about 2 by 2 by ½ in	1 piece	45	155	2	16	0	1
Shredded or grated, not pressed down.	1 cup	80	275	3	28	0	2
Filberts (hazelnuts), chopped (about 60 kernels).	1 cup	115	730	14	72	—	trace
Lentils, whole, cooked	1 cup	200	210	16	trace	40	0
Peanuts, roasted in oil, salted (whole, halves, chopped).	1 cup	144	840	37	72	—	0
Peanut butter	1 tbsp	16	95	4	8	—	0
Peas, split, dry, cooked	1 cup	200	230	16	1	80	—

Food	Measure						
Pecans, chopped or pieces (about 120 large halves).	1 cup	118	810	11	84	150	2
Pumpkin and squash kernels, dry, hulled.	1 cup	140	775	41	65	100	—
Sunflower seeds, dry, hulled	1 cup	145	810	35	69	70	—
Walnuts:							
Black:							
Chopped or broken kernels	1 cup	125	785	26	74	380	—
Ground (finely)	1 cup	80	500	16	47	240	—
Persian or English, chopped (about 60 halves).	1 cup	120	780	18	77	40	2

SUGARS AND SWEETS

Food	Measure						
Cake icings:							
Boiled, white:							
Plain	1 cup	94	295	1	0	0	0
With coconut	1 cup	166	605	3	13	0	0
Uncooked:							
Chocolate made with milk and butter.	1 cup	275	1,035	9	38	580	1
Creamy fudge from mix and water.	1 cup	245	830	7	16	trace	trace

SUGARS AND SWEETS Cont.

	Grams (gm.)	Cal.	Pro. (gm.)	Fat (gm.)	A (IU)	C (IU)
White	1 cup	319	1,200	2	21	860	trace
Candy:							
Caramels, plain or chocolate	1 oz	28	115	1	3	trace	trace
Chocolate:							
Milk, plain	1 oz	28	145	2	9	80	trace
Semisweet, small pieces (60 per oz)	1 cup or 6-oz pkg	170	860	7	61	30	0
Chocolate-coated peanuts	1 oz	28	160	5	12	trace	trace
Fondant, uncoated (mints, candy corn, other)	1 oz	28	105	trace	1	0	0
Fudge, chocolate, plain	1 oz	28	115	1	3	trace	trace
Gum drops	1 oz	28	100	trace	trace	0	0
Hard	1 oz	28	110	0	trace	0	0
Marshmallows	1 oz	28	90	1	trace	0	0
Chocolate-flavored beverage powders (about 4 heaping tsp per oz):							
With nonfat dry milk	1 oz	28	100	5	1	10	1
Without milk	1 oz	28	100	1	1	—	0
Honey, strained or extracted	1 tbsp	21	65	trace	0	0	trace

Food	Measure						
Jams and preserves	1 tbsp	20	55	trace	trace	trace	trace
	1 packet	14	40	trace	trace	trace	trace
Jellies	1 tbsp	18	50	trace	trace	trace	1
	1 packet	14	40	trace	trace	trace	1
Sirups:							
Chocolate-flavored sirup or topping:							
Thin type	1 fl oz or 2 tbsp	38	90	1	1	trace	0
Fudge type	1 fl oz or 2 tbsp	38	125	2	5	60	trace
Molasses, cane:							
Light (first extraction)	1 tbsp	20	50	—	—	—	—
Blackstrap (third extraction)	1 tbsp	20	45	—	—	—	—
Sorghum	1 tbsp	21	55	—	—	—	—
Table blends, chiefly corn, light and dark.	1 tbsp	21	60	0	0	0	0
Sugars:							
Brown, pressed down	1 cup	220	820	0	0	0	0
White:							
Granulated	1 cup	200	770	0	0	0	0
	1 tbsp	12	45	0	0	0	0
	1 packet	6	23	0	0	0	0
Powdered, sifted, spooned into cup.	1 cup	100	385	0	0	0	0

VEGETABLE AND VEGETABLE PRODUCTS

	Grams	Cal.	Pro. (gm.)	Fat (gm.)	A (IU)	C (IU)
Asparagus, green:						
Cooked, drained:						
Cuts and tips, 1½- to 2-in lengths:						
From raw .... 1 cup	145	30	3	trace	1,310	38
From frozen .... 1 cup	180	40	6	trace	1,530	41
Spears, ½-in diam. at base:						
From raw .... 4 spears	60	10	1	trace	540	16
From frozen .... 4 spears	60	15	2	trace	470	16
Canned, spears, ½-in diam. 4 spears at base.	80	15	2	trace	640	12
Beans:						
Lima, immature seeds, frozen, cooked, drained:						
Thick-seeded types (Fordhooks) .... 1 cup	170	170	10	trace	390	29
Thin-seeded types (baby limas) .... 1 cup	180	210	13	trace	400	22

Snap:						
Green:						
Cooked, drained:						
From raw (cuts and French style).	1 cup	125	30	2	trace	680	15
From frozen:						
Cuts	1 cup	135	35	2	trace	780	7
French style	1 cup	130	35	2	trace	690	9
Canned, drained solids (cuts).	1 cup	135	30	2	trace	630	5
Yellow or wax:						
Cooked, drained:						
From raw (cuts and French style).	1 cup	125	30	2	trace	290	16
From frozen (cuts)	1 cup	135	35	2	trace	140	8
Canned, drained solids (cuts).	1 cup	135	30	2	trace	140	7
Beans, mature. See Beans, dry and Blackeye peas, dry						
Bean sprouts (mung):						
Raw	1 cup	105	35	4	trace	20	20
Cooked, drained	1 cup	125	35	4	trace	30	8

VEGETABLES AND VEGETABLE PRODUCTS Cont.

		Grams	Cal.	Pro. (gm.)	Fat (gm.)	A (IU)	C (IU)
Beets:							
Cooked, drained, peeled:							
Whole beets, 2-in diam.	2 beets	100	30	1	trace	20	6
Diced or sliced	1 cup	170	55	2	trace	30	10
Canned, drained solids:							
Whole beets, small	1 cup	160	60	2	trace	30	5
Diced or sliced	1 cup	170	65	2	trace	30	5
Beet greens, leaves and stems, cooked, drained.	1 cup	145	25	2	trace	7,400	22
Blackeye peas, immature seeds, cooked and drained:							
From raw	1 cup	165	180	13	1	580	28
From frozen	1 cup	170	220	15	1	290	15
Broccoli, cooked, drained:							
From raw:							
Stalk, medium size	1 stalk	180	45	6	1	4,500	162
Stalks cut into ½-in pieces	1 cup	155	40	5	trace	3,880	140
From frozen:							
Stalk, 4½ to 5 in long	1 stalk	30	10	1	trace	570	22
Chopped	1 cup	185	50	5	1	4,810	105

Brussels sprouts, cooked, drained:							
From raw, 7-8 sprouts (1¼- to 1½-in diam.).	1 cup	155	55	7	1	810	135
From frozen	1 cup	155	50	5	trace	880	126
Cabbage:							
Common varieties:							
Raw:							
Coarsely shredded or sliced	1 cup	70	15	1	trace	90	33
Finely shredded or chopped	1 cup	90	20	1	trace	120	42
Cooked, drained	1 cup	145	30	2	trace	190	48
Red, raw, coarsely shredded or sliced.	1 cup	70	20	1	trace	30	43
Savoy, raw, coarsely shredded or sliced.	1 cup	70	15	2	trace	140	39
Cabbage, celery (also called pe-tsai or wongbok), raw 1-in pieces.	1 cup	75	10	1	trace	110	19
Cabbage, white mustard (also called bokchoy or pakchoy), cooked, drained.	1 cup	170	25	2	trace	5,270	26

VEGETABLES AND VEGETABLE PRODUCTS Cont.		Grams	Cal. (gm.)	Pro. (gm.)	Fat (gm.)	A (IU)	C (IU)
Carrots:							
Raw, without crowns and tips, scraped:							
Whole, 7½ by 1⅛ in, or strips, 2½ to 3 in long.	1 carrot or 18 strips	72	30	1	trace	7,930	6
Grated	1 cup	110	45	1	trace	12,100	9
Cooked (crosswise cuts), drained	1 cup	155	50	1	trace	16,280	9
Canned:							
Sliced, drained solids	1 cup	155	45	1	trace	23,250	3
Strained or junior (baby food)	1 oz (1¾ to 2 tbsp)	28	10	trace	trace	3,690	1
Cauliflower:							
Raw, chopped	1 cup	115	31	3	trace	70	90
Cooked, drained:							
From raw (flower buds)	1 cup	125	30	3	trace	80	69
From frozen (flowerets)	1 cup	180	30	3	trace	50	74
Celery, Pascal type, raw:							
Stalk, large outer, 8 by 1½ in, at root end.	1 stalk	40	5	trace	trace	110	4

Pieces, diced	1 cup	120	1	trace	320	11
Collards, cooked, drained: From raw (leaves without stems)	1 cup	190	7	1	14,820	144
From frozen (chopped)	1 cup	170	5	1	11,560	56
Corn, sweet: Cooked, drained: From raw, ear 5 by 1¾ in	1 ear	140	2	1	[43]310	7
From frozen: Ear, 5 in long	1 ear	229	4	1	[43]440	9
Kernels	1 cup	165	5	1	[43]580	8
Canned: Cream style	1 cup	256	5	2	[43]840	13
Whole kernel: Vacuum pack	1 cup	210	5	1	[43]740	11
Wet pack, drained solids	1 cup	165	4	1	[43]580	7
Cowpeas. See Black eye peas						
Cucumber slices, ⅛ in thick (large, 2⅛-in diam.; small, 1¾-in diam.): With peel	6 large or 8 small slices	28	trace	trace	70	3
Without peel	6½ large or 9 small pieces	28	trace	trace	trace	3

[43]Based on yellow varieties. For white varieties, value is trace.

VEGETABLES AND VEGETABLE PRODUCTS Cont.

		Grams	Cal.	Pro. (gm.)	Fat (gm.)	A (IU)	C (IU)
Dandelion greens, cooked, drained	1 cup	105	35	2	1	12,290	19
Endive, curly (including escarole), raw, small pieces.	1 cup	50	10	1	trace	1,650	5
Garlic	1 clove	3	4	.2	trace	trace	trace
Kale, cooked, drained:							
From raw (leaves without stems and midribs).	1 cup	110	45	5	1	9,130	102
From frozen (leaf style)	1 cup	130	40	4	1	10,660	49
Lettuce, raw:							
Butterhead, as Boston types:							
Head, 5-in diam.	1 head	220	25	2	trace	1,580	13
Leaves	1 outer or 2 inner or 3 heart leaves.	15	trace	trace	trace	150	1
Crisphead, as Iceberg:							
Head, 6-in diam.	1 head	567	70	5	1	1,780	32
Wedge, 1/4 of head	1 wedge	135	20	1	trace	450	8
Pieces, chopped or shredded	1 cup	55	5	trace	trace	180	3
Looseleaf (bunching varieties including romaine or cos), chopped or shredded pieces.	1 cup	55	10	1	trace	1,050	10

Food	Measure						
Mushrooms, raw, sliced or chopped	1 cup	70	20	trace	2	trace	2
Mustard greens, without stems and midribs, cooked, drained.	1 cup	140	30	3	1	8,120	67
Okra pods, 3 by ⅝ in, cooked	10 pods	106	30	2	trace	520	21
Onions:							
Mature:							
Raw:							
Chopped	1 cup	170	65	3	trace	[44]trace	17
Sliced	1 cup	115	45	2	trace	[44]trace	12
Cooked (whole or sliced), drained.	1 cup	210	60	3	trace	[44]trace	15
Young green, bulb (⅜ in diam.) and white portion of top.	6 onions	30	15	trace	trace	trace	8
Parsley, raw, chopped	1 tbsp	4	trace	trace	trace	300	6
Parsnips, cooked (diced or 2-in lengths).	1 cup	155	100	2	1	50	16
Peas, green:							
Canned:							
Whole, drained solids	1 cup	170	150	8	1	1,170	14
Strained (baby food)	1 oz (1¾ to 2 tbsp)	28	15	1	trace	140	3

[44]Value based on white-fleshed varieties. For yellow-fleshed varieties, value in International Units (IU) is 70 (raw chopped). 50 (raw sliced), and 80 (cooked).

VEGETABLES AND VEGETABLE PRODUCTS *Cont.*

	Grams	Cal.	Pro. (gm.)	Fat (gm.)	A (IU)	C (IU)
Frozen, cooked, drained	1 cup	160	110	8	trace	960	21
Peppers, hot, red, without seeds, dried (ground chili powder, added seasonings).	1 tsp	2	5	trace	trace	1,300	trace
Peppers, sweet (about 5 per lb, whole), stem and seeds removed:							
Raw	1 pod	74	15	1	trace	310	94
Cooked, boiled, drained	1 pod	73	15	1	trace	310	70
Potatoes, cooked:							
Baked, peeled after baking (about 2 per lb, raw).	1 potato	156	145	4	trace	trace	31
Boiled (about 3 per lb, raw):							
Peeled after boiling	1 potato	137	105	3	trace	trace	22
Peeled before boiling	1 potato	135	90	3	trace	trace	22
French-fried, strip, 2 to 3½ in long:							
Prepared from raw	10 strips	50	135	2	7	trace	11
Frozen, oven heated	10 strips	50	110	2	4	trace	11

Hashed brown, prepared from frozen.	1 cup	155	345	3	18	trace	12
Mashed, prepared from— Raw:							
Milk added	1 cup	210	135	4	2	40	21
Milk and butter added	1 cup	210	195	4	9	360	19
Dehydrated flakes (without milk), water, milk, butter, and salt added.	1 cup	210	195	4	7	270	11
Potato chips, 1¾ by 2½ in oval cross section.	10 chips	20	115	1	8	trace	3
Potato salad, made with cooked salad dressing.	1 cup	250	250	7	7	350	28
Pumpkin, canned	1 cup	245	80	2	1	15,680	12
Radishes, raw (prepackaged) stem ends, rootlets cut off.	4 radishes	18	5	trace	trace	trace	5
Sauerkraut, canned, solids and liquid.	1 cup	235	40	2	trace	120	33
Southern peas. See Blackeye peas							
Spinach:							
Raw, chopped	1 cup	55	15	2	trace	4,460	28
Cooked, drained: From raw	1 cup	180	40	5	1	14,580	50

VEGETABLES AND VEGETABLE PRODUCTS *Cont.*

		Grams	Cal.	Pro. (gm.)	Fat (gm.)	A (IU)	C (IU)
From frozen:							
Chopped	1 cup	205	45	6	1	16,200	39
Leaf	1 cup	190	45	6	1	15,390	53
Canned, drained solids	1 cup	205	50	6	1	16,400	29
Squash, cooked:							
Summer (all varieties), diced, drained.	1 cup	210	30	2	trace	820	21
Winter (all varieties), baked, mashed.	1 cup	205	130	4	1	8,610	27
Sweet potatoes:							
Cooked (raw, 5 by 2 in; about 2½ per lb):							
Baked in skin, peeled	1 potato	114	160	2	1	9,230	25
Boiled in skin, peeled	1 potato	151	170	3	1	11,940	26
Candied, 2½ by 2-in piece	1 piece	105	175	1	3	6,620	11
Canned:							
Solid pack (mashed)	1 cup	255	275	5	1	19,890	36
Vacuum pack, piece 2¾ by 1 in.	1 piece	40	45	1	trace	3,120	6

Tomatoes:							
Raw, 2⅗-in diam. (3 per 12 oz pkg.).	1 tomato	135	25	1	trace	1,110	28
Canned, solids and liquid	1 cup	241	50	2	trace	2,170	41
Tomato catsup	1 cup	273	290	5	1	3,820	41
	1 tbsp	15	15	trace	trace	210	2
Tomato juice, canned:							
Cup	1 cup	243	45	2	trace	1,940	39
Glass (6 fl oz)	1 glass	182	35	2	trace	1,460	29
Turnips, cooked, diced	1 cup	155	35	1	trace	trace	34
Turnip greens, cooked, drained:							
From raw (leaves and stems)	1 cup	145	30	3	trace	8,270	68
From frozen (chopped)	1 cup	165	40	4	trace	11,390	31
Vegetables, mixed, frozen, cooked	1 cup	182	115	6	1	9,010	15

MISCELLANEOUS ITEMS

Baking powders for home use:							
Sodium aluminum sulfate:							
With monocalcium phosphate monohydrate.	1 tsp	3.0	5	trace	trace	0	0

MISCELLANEOUS ITEMS Cont.

	Grams	Cal.	Pro. (gm.)	Fat (gm.)	A (IU)	C (IU)
With monocalcium phosphate monohydrate, calcium sulfate.	2.9	5	trace	trace	0	0
Straight phosphate .... 1 tsp	3.8	5	trace	trace	0	0
Low sodium .... 1 tsp	4.3	5	trace	trace	0	0
Barbecue sauce .... 1 cup	250	230	4	17	900	13
Beverages, alcoholic:						
Beer .... 12 fl oz	360	150	1	0	—	—
Gin, rum, vodka, whisky:						
80-proof .... 1½-fl oz jigger	42	95	—	—	—	—
86-proof .... 1½-fl oz jigger	42	105	—	—	—	—
90-proof .... 1½-fl oz jigger	42	110	—	—	—	—
Wines:						
Dessert .... 3½-fl oz glass	103	140	trace	0	—	—
Table .... 3½-fl oz glass	102	85	trace	0	—	—
Beverages, carbonated, nonalcoholic:						
Carbonated water .... 12 fl oz	366	0	0	0	0	0
Cola type .... 12 fl oz	369	145	0	0	0	0

Food	Amount						
Fruit-flavored sodas and Tom Collins mixer.	12 fl oz	372	170	0	0	0	0
Ginger ale	12 fl oz	366	115	0	0	0	0
Root beer	12 fl oz	370	150	0	0	0	0
Chili powder. See Peppers, hot, red							
Chocolate:							
Bitter or baking	1 oz	28	145	3	15	20	0
Semisweet, see Candy, chocolate							
Gelatin, dry	1, 7-g envelope	7	25	6	trace	—	—
Gelatin dessert prepared with gelatin dessert powder and water.	1 cup	240	140	4	0	—	—
Mustard, prepared, yellow	1 tsp or individual serving pouch or cup.	5	5	trace	trace	—	—
Olives, pickled, canned:							
Green	4 medium or 3 extra large or 2 giant.	16	15	trace	2	40	
Ripe, Mission	3 small or 2 large	10	15	trace	2	10	
Pickles, cucumber:							
Dill, medium, whole, 3¾ in long, 1¼-in diam.	1 pickle	65	5	trace	trace	70	

MISCELLANEOUS ITEMS *Cont.*

	Grams	Cal.	Pro. (gm.)	(gm.)		
Fresh-pack, slices, 1½-in diam., ¼ in thick.	2 slices	15	10	trace	tra	
Sweet, gherkin, small, whole, about 2½ in long, ¾-in diam.	1 pickle	15	20	trace	trace	
Relish, finely chopped, sweet	1 tbsp	15	20	trace	trace	
Popsicle, 3-fl oz size	1 popsicle	95	70	0	0	
Soups:						
Canned, condensed:						
Prepared with equal volume of milk:						
Cream of chicken	1 cup	245	180	7	10	610
Cream of mushroom	1 cup	245	215	7	14	250	1
Tomato	1 cup	250	175	7	7	1,200	15
Prepared with equal volume of water:						
Bean with pork	1 cup	250	170	8	6	650	3
Beef broth, bouillon, consomme.	1 cup	240	30	5	0	trace	—
Beef noodle	1 cup	240	65	4	3	50	trace

		245	80	2	3	880	—
Clam chowder, Manhattan type (with tomatoes, without milk).	1 cup						
Cream of chicken	1 cup	240	95	3	6	410	trace
Cream of mushroom	1 cup	240	135	2	10	70	trace
Minestrone	1 cup	245	105	5	3	2,350	—
Split pea	1 cup	245	145	9	3	440	1
Tomato	1 cup	245	90	2	3	1,000	12
Vegetable beef	1 cup	245	80	5	2	2,700	—
Vegetarian	1 cup	245	80	2	2	2,940	—
Dehydrated:							
Bouillon cube, ½ in	1 cube	4	5	1	trace	—	—
Mixes:							
Unprepared:							
Onion	1½-oz pkg	43	150	6	5	30	6
Prepared with water:							
Chicken noodle	1 cup	240	55	2	1	50	trace
Onion	1 cup	240	35	1	1	trace	2
Tomato vegetable with noodles.	1 cup	240	65	1	1	480	5
Vinegar, cider	1 tbsp	15	trace	trace	0	—	—

MISCELLANEOUS ITEMS Cont.

	Grams	Cal.	Pro. (gm.)	Fat (gm.)	A (IU)	C (IU)
White sauce, medium, with enriched flour.	1 cup	250	405	10	31	1,150	2
Yeast:							
Baker's, dry active	1 pkg	7	20	3	trace	trace	trace
Brewer's, dry	1 tbsp	8	25	3	trace	trace	trace

CHAPTER SIXTEEN

SPECIAL-INTEREST RECIPES

Once you start eating and cooking with the Lifelong Anti-Cancer Diet in mind, a whole world of food ideas and recipes are available to you.

Instead of that same fried fish or shellfish, you can have fish poached in a court bouillon. There are many interesting ways to prepare cruciferous vegetables, beans, and whole grains. Vegetables can be presented as a main dish or combined with a small amount of meat to create dishes high in nutrients, low in fat, and full of flavor.

You may think you'll never like certain of the foods that are recommended. But finding ways to prepare them so you *will* like them is not difficult and is one of the pleasures of creative cooking. Take kale, for example. It makes a terrific addition to such Japanese dishes as sukiyaki, shabu-shabu, and clear soups. Pureed cooked kale combines with mashed potatoes for a different vegetable dish. Kale may be cooked in an Italian manner, somewhat similar to the way escarole or spinach is prepared; a recipe is given in this chapter. Kale may be used instead of sorrel, spinach, or watercress in soups or sauces. Parboiled kale, chopped, can be added to stuffings for breast of veal, or any stuffed lamb dish.

The following is only a brief selection of additional recipes that incorporate these nutritional ideas as guide-

217

lines. You'll discover many more; there's no lack of variety or imagination on the Lifelong Anti-Cancer Diet.

EASY BEAN PUREE

1 16-ounce can white cannellini beans
1 clove garlic, pressed
½ cup chicken broth or 2 tablespoons butter or margarine

Salt and freshly ground white pepper to taste

Pour cannellini beans into a colander. Drain, and rinse with water. Drain again.

Using a food mill or a food processor, puree beans. Spoon beans into a saucepan and add all other ingredients. Stir to combine and heat before serving.

Serves: 4

WESTERN-STYLE BEANS

1 cup pinto beans or red kidney beans
Water
1 onion
1 teaspoon salt
1 small green chili pepper, seeded and chopped (optional)
2 medium tomatoes, peeled and coarsely chopped

½ teaspoon ground cinnamon
1 onion, chopped
Juice of ½ lemon
Salt and freshly ground black pepper to taste

Place beans in a large saucepan, add water to cover, and bring to a boil. Cook beans for 2 minutes, remove from heat, cover, and allow to stand for 1 hour.

Add onion and salt to pot, and continue cooking until beans are tender, about 1 to 1½ hours, depending on the age of the beans. Add more water to saucepan, if necessary.

Drain all but 1 cup of cooking liquid from beans. Combine beans, 1 cup of bean cooking liquid, and all other ingredients. Cook, covered, for 30 minutes, until sauce is reduced and thick.

Serves: 4–6

BROCCOLI PUREE

1 bunch broccoli, cooked, cut into large pieces
2 tablespoons butter or margarine, softened

Salt and freshly ground black pepper to taste

Using a food processor or food mill, puree broccoli coarsely. Add all other ingredients, and combine thoroughly.

Heat before serving.
Serves: 4

BRUSSELS SPROUTS WITH CHEESE

1 quart brussels sprouts (about 1½ pounds)
½ cup grated Parmesan cheese

½ cup bread crumbs
1 tablespoon melted butter or margarine

Wash brussels sprouts, and trim off any wilted outside leaves. Cut a small, shallow cross in the bottom of each brussels sprout.

Cook brussels sprouts in boiling water to cover for 15 to 20 minutes until brussels sprouts are just tender. Do not overcook. Drain sprouts and reserve.

Combine grated cheese and bread crumbs, mixing thoroughly. Roll brussels sprouts in cheese-crumb mixture, and place in a single layer on a nonstick baking pan.

Drizzle melted butter over brussels sprouts, and bake in a preheated 400 degree oven for 10 to 15 minutes, or until brussels sprouts are brown.

Serves: 6

BRUSSELS SPROUTS WITH SESAME SEEDS

1 quart brussels sprouts (about 1½ pounds)
2 cups beef or vegetable broth

Salt and freshly ground black pepper to taste
2 tablespoons sesame seeds, lightly toasted

Wash brussels sprouts, and trim off any wilted outside leaves. Cut a small, shallow cross in the bottom of each brussels sprout.

Parboil brussels sprouts in boiling water for 5 to 10 minutes, until almost tender. Drain brussels sprouts and reserve.

Heat broth in a sauce pan, and bring to a simmer. Add brussels sprouts and seasonings. Cover, and cook an additional 10 to 15 minutes, or until tender. Most of the broth will have been absorbed by the brussels sprouts. Drain sprouts, if necessary, and toss with sesame seeds.

Serves: 6

BULGUR PILAF

2 tablespoons butter or
margarine
1 small onion, chopped
1 cup sliced
mushrooms
1 small green pepper,
seeded, and chopped
1 tablespoon chopped
parsley

1 cup bulgur
¼ teaspoon ground
cumin
Salt and freshly ground
black pepper to taste
2 cups beef or chicken
or vegetable broth or
bouillon

Heat butter in a large skillet. Add onion, mushrooms, and green pepper, and cook, stirring, until onion and green pepper are translucent, about 3 to 5 minutes.

Add parsley and bulgur to skillet, and continue sautéing, stirring until bulgur is golden.

Add seasonings and broth or bouillon. Cover, and bring to a boil. Reduce heat, and simmer for 15 to 20 minutes, or until bulgur is tender and liquid is absorbed.

Serves: 4

CABBAGE STUFFED WITH RICE AND RAISINS

1 large head cabbage
1 tablespoon vegetable oil
1 small onion, grated
1 cup brown rice
2 cups vegetable broth or bouillon
3 tablespoons raisins
¼ cup toasted sunflower seeds
Salt and freshly ground black pepper to taste

1 tablespoon oil
1 tablespoon all-purpose flour or whole wheat flour
2 cups tomato sauce
2 cups water
1 teaspoon sugar
¼ teaspoon red pepper flakes (optional)

Parboil cabbage for 10 to 15 minutes in boiling water. Drain and allow to cool.

Heat oil in a large skillet. Sauté onion in oil for 3 minutes, stirring. Add rice, and sauté another 2 minutes. Add vegetable broth, raisins, sunflower seeds, and seasonings. Bring to a simmer, cover, and cook for 30 minutes.

Separate cabbage into individual leaves. Spoon 2 tablespoons of rice filling on each leaf, being careful to tuck in ends as you roll each cabbage leaf.

To prepare sauce, use a large casserole or dutch oven. Heat 1 tablespoon of oil and add flour. Cook, stirring, for 2 minutes. Gradually stir in tomato sauce and water. Cook, stirring, and add sugar and red pepper flakes, if you wish. Bring sauce to a simmer, and using a large spoon, carefully place cabbage rolls in casserole.

Cover, and simmer over low heat for 45 minutes

to 1 hour, or until cabbage and rice are completely cooked

Serves: 6–8

Note: This Rice and Raisin stuffing may also be used for green peppers.

CAULIFLOWER APPETIZER WITH DILL-YOGURT DIP

1 head cauliflower
1 cup low-fat yogurt
3 tablespoons low-calorie mayonnaise
¼ teaspoon white pepper

Dash paprika
2 tablespoons chopped fresh dill

Separate cauliflower into small flowerets, and place on a serving platter.

Combine all other ingredients, mixing thoroughly, and spoon into a small bowl. Place bowl containing dip beside cauliflower.

Serves: 6–8

CAULIFLOWER AND SWISS CHEESE

1 head cauliflower, cut into large flowerets
½ cup grated Swiss cheese
½ cup bread crumbs
⅛ teaspoon freshly ground white pepper (optional)

1 tablespoon melted butter or margarine
1 tablespoon chopped parsley

Wash cauliflower and separate into large flowerets for quicker cooking.

Cook cauliflower in boiling water to cover, for 10 to 20 minutes, or until vegetable is just tender. Do not overcook. Drain cauliflower and place flowerets on a nonstick baking pan.

Combine cheese, bread crumbs, and seasonings, and mix thoroughly. Spoon over cauliflower, and drizzle melted butter over all.

Bake in a preheated 400-degree oven for 5 to 10 minutes, or until cauliflower is hot, and topping has browned slightly.

Serves: 4–6

COURT BOUILLON

Instead of deep-frying fish, or sautéing or broiling with butter or oil, poach fish and shellfish in a court bouillon—a flavorful, low-fat alternative.

2 stalks celery	10 black peppercorns
6 sprigs parsley	¼ teaspoon thyme
1 bay leaf	1 medium onion
1 cup white vinegar	Bones and head of fish
2 quarts water	(optional)

Combine all ingredients in a large saucepan, and bring to a simmer. Cook, uncovered for 20 minutes. Strain before using.

To poach fish or shellfish, bring court bouillon to a boil before placing fish or shellfish into liquid.

GREEN PEPPERS STUFFED WITH CHICKPEAS AND RICE

6 medium green peppers

1 cup cooked chickpeas, pureed

2 cups cooked brown or white rice

2 tomatoes finely chopped

1 tablespoon vegetable oil

1 medium onion, grated

2 tablespoons chopped parsley

Salt and freshly ground black pepper to taste

2 cups vegetable broth or bouillon

Carefully cut tops off green peppers. Remove seeds from peppers and reserve peppers and tops.

Combine all other ingredients, except for vegetable broth, mix thoroughly, and stuff mixture into green peppers. Cover peppers with reserved tops and place in a dutch oven. Pour vegetable broth around peppers, and add enough water so that peppers are half-covered.

Cook for about 1 hour, or until peppers are tender. Remove peppers from dutch oven and place on a platter. Refrigerate, and serve cold.

Serves: 6

KALE, ITALIAN-STYLE

1 bunch kale (about ½ pound)
1 tablespoon olive oil
1 clove garlic, finely chopped
1 teaspoon pignolia nuts, also known as pine nuts (optional)

Salt and freshly ground black pepper to taste

Wash kale, and snap off stems and discard.

Steam, or cook kale in water to cover, for approximately 5 to 10 minutes, or until vegetable is tender but not limp. Drain and reserve.

Heat olive oil in a nonstick pan. Add garlic, and pignolia nuts if desired. Cook over low heat, stirring, until garlic and nuts are very lightly browned.

Add kale to olive oil, and cook another 2 to 3 minutes, stirring to combine, until kale is hot.

Serves: 2–3

STUFFED ZUCCHINI

⅓ cup yellow split peas
1 small onion, grated
½ pound ground veal
½ cup cooked white or brown rice
4 tablespoons chopped fresh dill
Salt and freshly ground black pepper to taste

¼ teaspoon ground cinnamon
6 medium zucchini, scraped
2 cups tomato sauce

Cook split peas until soft, about 30 minutes. Drain, and spoon into a large bowl. Combine split peas with onion, ground veal, cooked rice, dill, and seasonings. Mix thoroughly, and reserve.

Parboil zucchini in boiling water until barely tender, about ten minutes. Drain, and allow to cool.

Cut zucchini in half. Scoop out centers and discard. Fill zucchini halves with split pea and veal mixture. Pour tomato sauce into a baking dish, and place zucchini halves on top.

Bake in a preheated 350-degree oven for 45 minutes, or until zucchini is tender and meat is cooked.

Serves: 6

CARROT PUREE

2 pounds carrots, scraped, cut into pieces, and cooked
1 tablespoon butter, or margarine

½ cup chicken broth
Salt and freshly ground white pepper to taste
¼ teaspoon ground coriander

Using a food processor or food mill, puree carrots coarsely. Add all other ingredients, and combine thoroughly.

Heat before serving.

Serves: 4

INDEX

228

vitamin A in foods listed (*cont.*)
  in cheeses, 143–45
  in cherries, 167
  in chicken and chicken products, 164
  in chili con carne, 160
  in chop suey, 160
  in citrus fruits, 168–71, 173, 175
  in cranberries and cranberry products, 167
  in cream and cream-type products, 145–46
  in custards and puddings, 151
  in dates, 167
  in doughnuts, 187
  in eggs, 152
  in fish and shellfish, 156–58
  in flours, 181, 194–95
  in fruits and fruit products, 165–75
  in gelatins, 213
  in grains and grain prducts, 176–81, 192, 194–95
  in honey, 198
  in jams and jellies, 199
  in lamb, 160–61
  in legumes, 195–96
  in liver, 160
  in luncheon meat, 161
  in margarine, 153–54
  in meat and meat products, 158–62
  in milk and milk products, 142–51
  in nuts and seeds, 195–97
  in pancakes, 189
  in pasta, 188, 189, 193–94
  in pastry, 187, 194
  in pies, 189–91
  in pizza, 191
  in popcorn, 191
  in pretzels, 192
  in raisins, 174–75
  in relishes and pickles, 213–14

  in rice and rice products, 192
  in salad and cooking oils, 154–55
  in salad dressings, 155–56
  in sausages, 162–63
  in shortenings, 153
  in sirups and toppings, 199
  in soups, 214–15
  in sugars, 199
  in turkey and turkey products, 164
  in veal, 163
  in vinegar, 215
  in yeast, 216
  in yogurt, 151
vitamin B complex, 54
vitamin C
  in anti-cancer diet, 9, 26, 53–54, 73–76
  and copper, 56
  in fruits and vegetables, 39, 40, 46
  megadoses of, 54
  nutritional role of, 53–54
vitamin C in foods listed:
  in bacon, 158
  in bagel, 176
  in baking powders, 211–12
  in barbeque sauce, 212
  in beef and beef products, 158–60
  in berries, 167, 175
  in beverages: alcoholic, 212; carbonated, 212–13
  in breads and bread products, 176–79, 192–93
  in butter, 152–53
  in cakes and cookies, 182–86
  in candy and cake icings, 197–98
  in cereals, 179–91
  in cheeses, 143–45
  in cherries, 167
  in chicken and chicken products, 164
  in chili con carne, 160

Other SIGNET Books of Special Interest

Buy them at your local

bookstore or use coupon

on next page for ordering.

SIGNET and MENTOR Books of Related Interest